THE
HERBAL
COMPANION

The Essential Guide to Using Herbs for
Your Health and Well-Being

MARCUS A. WEBB

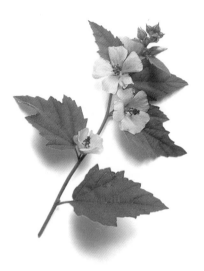

I dedicate this book to my wife, Mhairi. I seem to take on major projects just as new additions to our family are due. When our first baby, Cameron, was born I was in the middle of finishing an academic thesis, and just as our second baby was due, I decided to undertake the writing of this book. Mhairi, without your support and understanding neither of these projects would have been possible.

Acknowledgments
I owe special thanks to: Sue Wallander of Enzymatic Therapy (USA), Melanie Cook of Enzymatic Therapy (UK), Jen and Janyn Tan of Bioforce (UK), Pamela Cranston, Jan de Vries and Kathy Steer of Quintet Publishing.
A special thanks goes to Terry Griffiths for his introduction to Quintet Publishing and to my wife, Mhairi, for reading through the final copy so carefully and correcting my dreadful spelling!

THE
HERBAL
COMPANION

The Essential Guide to Using Herbs for
Your Health and Well-Being

MARCUS A. WEBB

≡ People's Medical Society®

Allentown, Pennsylvania

A QUINTET BOOK

First published in the United States in 1997 by the People's Medical Society

Library of Congress Cataloging-in-Publication Data
Webb, Marcus A.
The herbal companion: the essential guide to using herbs for your health and well-being/by Marcus A. Webb.
p. cm.
Includes index
ISBN 1-882606-34-5
1. Herbs – Therapeutic use. 2. Herb gardening. 3. Herbs – utilization. I. Title. RM666.H33W378 1997 615'. 321--dc21 97-8031 CIP

The People's Medical Society is a nonprofit consumer health organization dedicated to the principles of better, more responsive and less expensive medical care. Organized in 1983, the People's Medical Society puts previously unavailable medical information into the hands of consumers so that they can make informed decisions about their own health care. Membership in the People's Medical Society is $20 a year and includes a subscription to the *People's Medical Society Newsletter.* For information, write to the People's Medical Society, 462 Walnut Street, Allentown, PA 18102, or call 610-770-1670. This and other People's Medical Society Publications are available for quality purchase at discount. Contact the People's Medical Society for details.

This book was designed and produced by
Quintet Publishing Limited
6 Blundell Street
London N7 9BH

1234567890 First printing, September 1997

Typeset in Great Britain by
Central Southern Typesetters, Eastbourne
Manufactured in Singapore by Eray Scan Pte Ltd.
Printed in China by Leefung-Asco Printers Ltd.

The Publisher would like to thank the following for providing photographs and for permission to reproduce copyright material.
A–Z Botanical Collection: pp 11, 32, 50, 51, 52, 56, 57, 64, 65, 67, 75, 77, 78, 79, 82, 84, 86, 87, 89, 91, 94, 95, 97, 98, 99, 101, 103, 106, 107, 112, 115, 117, 122, 123, 124, 127, 128, 129, 136, 145, 146, 150, 154
Garden Matters: pp 9, 15, 16, 49, 85, 55, 71, 80, 88, 96, 108, 120, 121, 135, 143, 148, 155

CONTENTS

FOREWORD

It is with the greatest pleasure that I am writing the foreword to this book.

I have known Marcus for many years and have been impressed by the tremendous effort that he has taken to study all kinds of medicine. Not only has he developed knowledge in the orthodox way of medicine, but he has also developed knowledge in all the alternative fields.

Orthodox medicine, which I studied many years ago, has done a wonderful job, and it is with the greatest respect that I see how it has developed scientifically. It is, however, very important in today's society, where all kinds of health problems arise, to remember the three forms of energy that we live by—the food we eat, the water we drink and the air we breathe—so that bridges can be built between orthodox and alternative medicine to arrive at a complementary system, which will help alleviate human suffering. After all, both disciplines are working very hard toward the same purpose. Orthodox medicine is the result of a technical revolution and has not been with us for long. Alternative medicine, on the other hand, has been here for as long as we can remember. It is encouraging that in nature, where everything is balanced, there are herbs that can work better than sophisticated drugs. Thus books such as this one are important to educate us in forms of medicine that can be taken without side effects. Marcus has done a lot to research this. He is always researching everything he does with his patients. That is why he is so successful as a lecturer and as a practitioner; he has feedback from his patients and can share the knowledge that he has gathered to help people to better health.

It was a fortunate occasion when Marcus and I met years ago and spoke about our shared interest. He was very interested in the knowledge that I learned from my former partner, Alfred Vogel, N.D., who was possibly regarded as one of the world's best-known herbalists and teachers of alternative medicine. Vogel taught me how to collect herbs, what methods had to be followed and how to extract their beneficial ingredients, and I was happy to share my own enthusiasm for the balance in nature with Marcus.

In this book Marcus Webb brings nature and the knowledge of herbal medicine a little closer to us, and not only does he help us understand these disciplines better, but he also encourages further development in a medical science that was forgotten for a time, but is now coming back to help fight illness and disease. I am convinced that this book will find a place on many bookshelves to enrich that original form of medicine.

Jan de Vries, D.ho.med., N.D., M.R.N., D.O., M.R.O., D.Ac., M.B.Ac.A.

Auchenkyle Natural Medicine Clinic
Troon, Scotland
1997

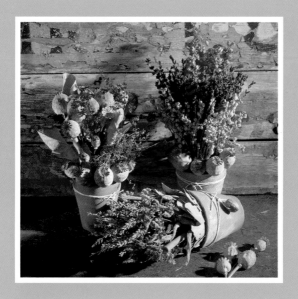

INTRODUCTION

Herbs can do far more for you than just garnish a finished dish: they can actually promote and protect your health. The use of traditional herbal remedies is a growth area in health care that is reflected in the 1994 sales figures for the United States of $1.6 billion. This enormous consumption of herbs is proof that something positive is gained by their use.

In 1995 the World Health Organization published figures that showed that more than 80 percent of the world's population used herbal medicines as their primary source of medication. This figure comes as no surprise when you consider that this form of medicine can be considered as original medicine, not alternative medicine.

The interest in herbal extracts has increased in the "developed" world as people look for safer ways to treat everyday illness and improve general health, while scientific interest is growing as the search for new therapeutic agents broadens. The potential discovery of, for example, a new anticancer drug extracted from a plant is a tempting and highly profitable reality. But as we purify the natural agents, we lose the very concept of herbal medicine that incorporates the whole plant, utilizing active agents and other essential factors that are naturally present in the herb. The whole plant extract will still be effective, but its action will be buffered by the cofactors present. Remove these and a pure "drug" is born with its undesirable side effects.

The aim of this book is to guide the interested reader through all aspects of herbs, from their growth through their medicinal uses. The discussions will, by the confines of this book, be brief but concise and easy to use. All the herbs in the directory are listed in Latin order. For quick reference there is a list of herbs with their common names on pages 46 and 47.

CAUTIONARY NOTE:

At all times it is recommended that you consult a health-care professional before embarking on a program of self-treatment. Herbal medicines are effective and safe when used in the correct circumstances. This book has been written to educate, and every effort has been made to make the book as accurate and as informative as possible, but the advice contained within is no replacement for professional guidance.

TRADITIONS AND HISTORY

In the Beginning

The use of herbs for the promotion of health can be dated back to the days of Hippocrates, who compiled a *materia medica* (a book containing information on herbs and their prescription) of more than 400 medicinal herbs during his lifetime (c. 460–370 B.C.). The works he left behind were soon built upon. The Greek philosopher Aristotle (c. 372–287 B.C.) wrote his monumental 10-volume compendium called *The History of Plants*, making him one of the most important contributors to our knowledge of botanical science.

Throughout history, herbs and their powers have played a very important part in our lives, so much so that the Egyptians immortalized their uses in stone tablets and tomb paintings.

Herb gardens first appeared during the eighth century.

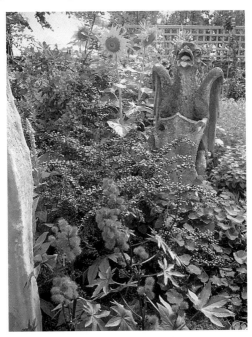

An apothecary's garden displaying different therapeutic herbs and flowers.

Monks grew medicinal herbs for treating of illness and for healing of wounds. The medieval opinion was that illness resulted from an imbalance in the four humors (phlegm, black and yellow bile, and blood) contained within the body. A popular treatment of the day was bloodletting. It was believed that this procedure allowed an excess of one of the humors to be drained away, and a preventive, quarterly bloodletting was performed on all monks living in the monasteries in an attempt to prevent an outbreak of disease. Herbs were frequently given to assist in the removal of excessive humors. Lavender was said to aid "pains in the head," violets were taken for diseases of the lung, and pennyroyal aided those with toothache. There were no physicians in the monasteries; the monks would train each other in treatment procedures and herbal applications. The information passed down from generation to generation firmly supported the effectiveness of herbal remedies and dictated the necessity for a well-stocked herb garden.

The first illustrated book on herbal preparations was written by the English herbalist and surgeon John Gerard. *The Herball, or Generall Historie of Plantes* was published in 1597 and gave comprehensive details of each plant including its origin, history, uses, methods of planting and the type of soil needed for each different species.

Unfortunately, one of herbal medicine's best-known advocates, Nicholas Culpeper, actually brought the practice of herbal cures into serious disrepute. Culpeper, who was an astrologer as well as a physician, classified the herbs according to astrological influences. The medical profession of Culpeper's day shunned him, since his teachings mixed magic and mystery with the old and accepted art of healing with herbs. Despite this, medicine came to acknowledge the power of plants in healing, and stronger extracts were purified to a point where only a few milligrams could exert a dramatic effect on the body.

The stage that conventional medicine has reached today is a long way from Hippocrates' original writings, even though the profession has taken his teachings and swears an oath in his name.

Important Influences on Herbal Medicine

It was not until the first century A.D. that the Roman physician Galen started to form a classification for the prescribing of herbal medicines based on the teachings of Hippocrates and formed his own classification for prescribing herbs. This was the first attempt to form a system of medicine that could be taught and followed by others, and it created a definite division between the physician and the traditional healers.

Inasmuch as this system of medicine helped to elevate herbal medicine, it did nothing to forward free thinking, and for approximately 1,500 years, the teachings of Galen were not challenged in Europe. It has been said that Galen did more to paralyze herbal medicine than anyone else, allowing the Galen-minded physicians to take over by prescribing herbs according to his teachings without actually considering the patient. In the days of the traditional herbalist, however, this would have been unthinkable because each patient was considered as an individual. Galen's teachings were, in fact, a direct contradiction to the faith the herbalists had in *vis medicatrix naturae*, the healing powers of nature.

During the sixteenth century Paracelsus challenged the teachings of Galen with his theory of the *Doctrine of Signatures*. This suggested that the physical characteristics of an herb indicated the area of the body that it was intended to treat. Paracelsus described illness as an external event (at this time syphilis and plague were widespread) for which the internal use of herbs was indicated.

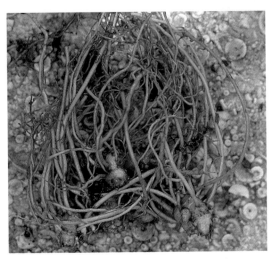

*Goldenseal (*Hydrastis canadensis*) originally grew in North America and became a popular remedy for relieving constipation.*

By 1785 herbs were being used for the treatment of many problems, one of which pushed forward the science of pharmacology dramatically. An English physician, William Withering, discovered that dropsy (heart failure) could be successfully treated with an extract of foxglove (*Digitalis*). This extract is still used to the present day in the form of the drug Digoxin.

The use of herbal medicine now appears to be turning full circle as scientists calculate that at least 328 new drugs could be developed from the plants of the tropical rain forests. Fresh interest is being generated in the healing powers of plants, an ancient wisdom that has stood the test of time.

The American Influence

The Americas offer many different climates and growing habitats for plants. Nearly all of the most important North American medicinal preparations originate from spices that grow native to the region.

As settlers adopted these remedies and discovered how effective they were for many different complaints, commercial growing was required to meet the demand. In 1838 the use of American herbal- and spice-based remedies spread to Europe, where their popularity soon grew. Remedies such as passionflower, goldenseal, witch hazel, sassafras, slippery elm and many other familiar preparations originally grew in North America.

From Central and South America the rain forest yielded, and is still yielding, a fascinating collection of plants with medicinal actions. As far back as the fourteenth century, a Florentine navigator, Amerigo Vespucci, discovered Colombian tribes chewing coca leaves, a practice stemming back to 2100 B.C. The alkaloid extracted from these leaves, cocaine, has become a valuable topical anesthetic as well as a lethal and addictive substance. Other commonly used plants from Central and South America include the chili pepper, Mexican yam, pawpaw, strychnine, boldo, allspice, Jamaican dogwood, vanilla and maize.

Conservation of this vital resource is essential, especially when cultivation for coca alone has accounted for the loss of more than 2 million acres (809,372 hectares) of rain forest in Peru since the early twentieth century.

GROWING HERBS

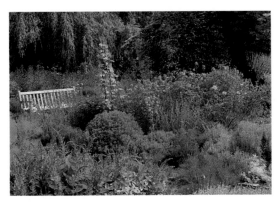

Careful planning can create wonderful visual effects in any garden or patch of land.

HERBS ARE NOT DIFFICULT to grow, and great satisfaction can be gotten from cultivating an herb garden or even growing just a pot of herbs.

Plant herbs outside when you can avoid having them damaged by excessive heat or cold. Most herbs enjoy a sunny location, but chives, feverfew, horseradish, lemon balm, mint, comfrey, ginger, violet, angelica, chervil, sweet woodruff, parsley and cicely are best planted in a shady place.

Selecting special herbs to plant in your herb garden will protect your crop from pests. If you plant rosemary and/or sage with your other herbs, you will prevent garden pests from destroying crops without needing to resort to chemical agents. This is important, especially if you are going to consume your produce.

Selecting the correct patch of land is important. Most herbs like at least six hours of light per day. Check the consistency of the soil: A sticky, muddy soil may need a little sand worked into it, but a stiff clay-based soil would benefit from some peat.

For your herbs to obtain optimal nutrition from the soil, make sure that the pH is slightly acidic to neutral (pH 6.5–7.9).

Herbs That Like Clay Soil

Angelica	Fennel
Chives	Lemon balm
Comfrey	Peppermint

Most garden centers will stock a pH testing kit. If your soil is too acidic, add some lime powder and if it is too alkaline, add some sulfur.

When choosing the most suitable herbs to grow, it will be necessary to select the best aspect, or exposure, of the ground. A southern exposure is considered the best, but the patch should be screened to the north and west by high-growing shrubs, conifers or a wall. Keeping the south and east aspects of the herb garden exposed is essential.

Water is a vital resource. Herbs should not be planted too far away from a hose or sprinkler. Herbs do respond well to rainwater, so storage is desirable for collecting this precious resource.

The best soils are generally loam-based, tending toward a sandy texture rather than a clay texture. A soil that has the characteristics of strength and lightness is perfect; this will make the best medium in which to grow any herbs irrespective of their species.

Herbs That Like a Dry Location

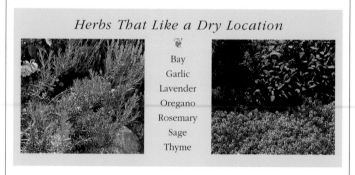

Bay
Garlic
Lavender
Oregano
Rosemary
Sage
Thyme

Herbs in the Garden

Growing herbs in a large garden will take some planning, and a visit to an established public herb garden will give you valuable ideas to bring home. An herb border is a good method of growing herbs for a kitchen garden. After seeing the plants growing in an established garden, you will get an accurate idea of how much certain species branch out and to what height they grow. For example, rosemary plants need to be spaced at least 3 feet (90 cm) apart, while fennel and marjoram need about 1 foot (30 cm) between each plant.

Herb borders make a very attractive addition to any garden as well as provide a great source of fresh herbs, but care must

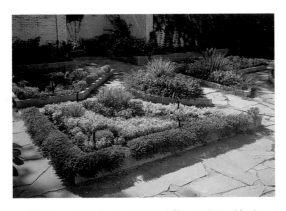

Herbs can look impressive in different shaped beds.

Shade-loving Herbs

Angelica	Horseradish
Chervil	Lemon balm
Chives	Parsley
Cicely	Peppermint
Comfrey	Sweet woodruff
Feverfew	Violet
Ginger	

be taken not to overplant the area. In a smaller garden the available space for planting is the important restricting factor, but with imagination there can be an infinite number of ways to create an impressive herbal display. Whether the beds are spread out in squares or circles depends on the location and number of herbs required.

Keep in mind that a kitchen garden needs to be close to the back door for ease of access. In this case it is likely that some of the area will be in shade for some of the day. Luckily there are some very useful herbs that thrive in the shade.

Herbs in Containers

Planting herbs in pots and containers is a very popular method, but they do need to be watered regularly and kept as near to the sunshine as possible. Container growing is also ideal if space is very tight. The pots may be piled up pyramid fashion if necessary. The number of herbs kept in a container

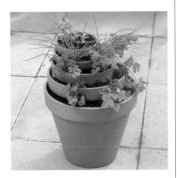

An unusual and attractive way of growing herbs is in a cascade.

depends, of course, on the size of the pot or container being used and its location. Don't forget that herbs spread out and some grow very fast, so allow plenty of room at the time of planting.

Window boxes planted with herbs are colorful and decorative. These can liven up any dull wall, and they do not have to be confined to a window ledge. The choice of

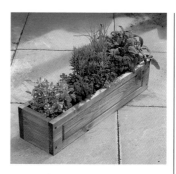

Window boxes are ideal placed on the kitchen window.

pots and containers is wide, but a classic wooden design is probably the best. If herbs are planted in a hanging wrought-iron container, the wind will have a dramatic drying effect on

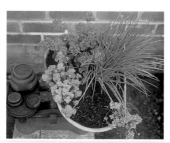

Herbs can be planted in any container such as a pair of old kitchen scales.

the soil. Some new designs of hanging baskets now have a built-in reservoir at the base of the container that can provide up to a week's water supply to the plants. This is a very good idea, especially in the hot summer months. Freestanding terra-cotta or glazed, decorative pottery containers look beautiful when planted, but they must be protected from frost,

which may crack them. Some are frost protected, making them the pots of choice where possible.

Herbs Suited to Containers

Basil	Oregano
Bay	Parsley
Chives	Peppermint
Feverfew	Rosemary
Hyssop	Sage
Lavender	Tarragon
Lemon balm	Thyme

A great way to start growing herbs is in a strawberry pot. This pot stands about 3 feet (90 cm) high, and it contains pockets around its circumference in which small plants can be planted. This method makes the most economical use of space and can be used in restricted areas such as a balcony, roof garden or outside the back door within reach of the kitchen.

When planting in a container, it is advisable to place some broken pots in the base of the pot to allow for drainage, then fill over with good-quality soil mixed with compost. Plant the herbs about 2 inches (5 cm) deep and press the soil down firmly. If planting seeds, scatter the seeds over the top of the soil, then cover with a little soil. Water well after planting.

Even in containers, some herbs such as fennel grow tall, whereas tarragon is naturally kept small by the restricted root space. Pruning will keep your container crop in check.

Essential Herbs to Grow

The planning of your herb garden is most important. Do you need herbs for cooking or are you looking to make medicinal remedies from your crop?

The commonly used culinary herbs are worth considering,

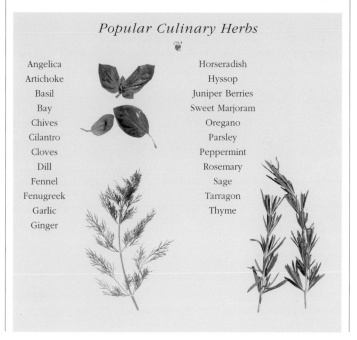

Popular Culinary Herbs

Angelica	Horseradish
Artichoke	Hyssop
Basil	Juniper Berries
Bay	Sweet Marjoram
Chives	Oregano
Cilantro	Parsley
Cloves	Peppermint
Dill	Rosemary
Fennel	Sage
Fenugreek	Tarragon
Garlic	Thyme
Ginger	

Popular Medicinal Herbs ❦		*Toxic Herbs* ❦
Caraway	Hyssop	Cowslip
Chamomile	Lavender	Foxglove
Cloves	Lemon balm	Glory lilies
Comfrey	Peppermint	Lily-of-the-valley
Echinacea	Rosemary	Madagascar periwinkle
Feverfew	Sage	Meadow saffron
Garlic	Thyme	Opium poppies
		Poke root

but grow only the ones that you use on a regular basis. Check which herbs are running low in the kitchen and plan to grow those first, as at least you know that they will be used. As you learn more about herbs and become more adventurous, you will be able to add new plants to your collection.

When choosing an herb crop to grow at home, don't forget that some are quite toxic and should be avoided whenever possible or at least positioned with great care, especially if you have young children or pets who may nibble the plants.

When and What to Plant

Garlic (*Allium sativum*) The bulbous root of the garlic is made up of 12–15 smaller cloves. The plant is grown by detaching the cloves and planting them. The soil should be light, dry and finely broken up. The cloves are planted 2½ inches (6 cm) apart and 1½ inches (4 cm) deep. They are best planted in early spring, and by the summer it is recommended that the leaves are tied in knots to prevent the stronger garlic plants from turning to flower.

The crop is harvested toward the end of summer. The roots are tied in bunches and hung in a dry room for later use.

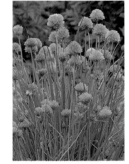

Chives (*Allium schoenoprasum*) Chives are readily grown by dividing the roots, either in the fall or spring, and will grow in any soil or situation. They should be repeatedly cut during the summer, which will cause successive leaves to grow through.

A small bed or border is easily managed and will continue to supply a productive crop for three to four years, after which a new planting should be cultivated.

Angelica (*Angelica archangelica*) Angelica is easily raised from seed that should be sown soon after it is gathered. It grows best in a moist soil and thrives exceedingly well by the side of a ditch. Though a biennial plant, it may be made to continue for several years by cutting down the flower stem before it goes to seed.

Celery (*Apium graveolens*) There are two varieties of celery: one with a hollow stalk and one with a solid stalk. The solid stalk is generally the preferred form to grow.

Celery must be sown at several different times in order to ensure a succession of plants throughout the year. The first sowing is made at the beginning of spring, in a sheltered border. The next planting can start at the end of spring in a moist border. By the middle of spring the plants of the first sowing will be ready for transplanting to nursery beds of rich earth, in which they can be planted 2 inches (5 cm) apart. Water is given, and the plants are shaded from direct sunlight for a few days. Toward the end of spring, the most mature plants can be transplanted into trenches for blanching. The normal method for transplanting and blanching follows:

Dig trenches 3–4 feet (90–120 cm) apart, 1 foot (30 cm) deep and 1 foot (30 cm) wide. Make sure that the soil at the base is fine and of good quality. The soil for celery needs to be moist, deep and rich, but still light. The earth dug from the trench is laid on either side ready to be drawn back in as wanted. The tops are cut off of the long leaves and any side roots, then the plants are placed in the base of the trench 2 inches (5 cm) apart. As they grow, the earth is drawn in toward them every 10 days. Care should be taken to do this in dry weather and not to cover the center of the plant with soil. When the plants rise above the ground level, the earth from around the edges of the trench will have become used up, so another trench needs to be dug between the rows for a supply of soil to continue the earthing up until the leaf stalks of the celery become blanched for 3 inches (8 cm). The last sowing can withstand a mild winter, and the soil into which the plants are transplanted should be dry. In severe winters, loose straw is thrown over the beds.

Horseradish (*Armoracia rusticana*) The soil for horseradish should be rich and deep. It is grown from cuttings of the knotty parts of the root that have one or two eyes present. They are planted in early spring, in rows, leaving 1 foot (30 cm) between each row. The cuttings are placed at a depth of at least 1 foot (30 cm). The roots are not used until the second year, when they are dug up as needed. The bed should last for four to five years.

Caraway (*Carum carvi*) The caraway is a biennial plant and should be sown soon after the seed is ripe in the fall. Thin out the plants during the next spring to within 4¾ inches (12 cm) apart. A moist soil suits the caraway plant best.

Artichoke (*Cynara scolymus*) Artichokes are grown by means of rooted slips or suckers taken off the main plant during spring. They like a light loam soil—cool, rich and deep but dry. In preparing for the crop, the soil should be dug in 3-foot (90 cm)-deep trenches and left to mature for a few days before planting. The plants should be placed 4 feet (120 cm) apart, and by the end of the season, a small crop of artichokes can be cut. In the second year the crop will be plentiful, and at the time the heads are gathered, by the fall, the whole stalks will be broken down close to the ground.

Hyssop (*Hyssopus officinalis*) a poor, dry soil is most suitable for hyssop. It may be grown in the spring months from seed, rooted slips or from cuttings.

Lavender (*Lavandula officinalis*) Lavender is grown from cuttings or young slips any time in the spring months. It should be planted in a dry, gravelly or poor soil.

Peppermint (*Mentha piperita*) Peppermint likes most soils and is readily grown from slips in the spring, by means of cuttings in the summer and by dividing the roots in the fall. Because peppermint plants are sometimes destroyed in a severe frost, it is advisable to cover them lightly with straw.

Sweet Marjoram (*Origanum majorana*) This herb is best grown from seed. Pot marjoram is propagated by cuttings and is hardy to withstand the winter. Winter sweet marjoram requires a sheltered border and a dry soil. It is a perennial plant and is propagated by dividing the roots in the fall.

Parsley (*Petroselinum crispum*) Parsley may be raised in shallow furrows on the edge of a border. The seeds may be sown in early spring.

Rosemary (*Rosmarinus officinalis*) Rosemary is easily grown from slips or cuttings in the spring. It should be planted in a dry soil in a shaded location.

Sage (*Salvia officinalis*) The lighter and poorer the soil, the better the sage will thrive. It is grown in the spring from slips and in the summer from cuttings. The cuttings should be up to 4¾ inches (12 cm) long, stripped of all the lower leaves and plunged nearly to the top in the earth. They must be well watered. The plants should be replaced every three to four years.

Thyme (*Thymus vulgaris*) Thyme grows best in a light, dry soil that has not been recently manured or fertilized. It is grown by parting the roots and planting the slips or by sowing the seeds in spring.

HARVESTING HERBS

Picking herbs tends to encourage new growth and stimulates the healthy development of the plant.

When picking the flowers it is best to take the bud just before it opens up, as most herbs reach their optimal flavor just prior to flowering. Perennial herbs can yield two or three good crops during their growing seasons, but it is best to give them one year to get established before harvesting. When collecting from perennials, it is important not to cut into the woody growth. For annuals it is possible to cut the crop to 4 inches (10 cm) from the soil twice during the growing season with a final harvesting just before the first frost.

If you wish to collect the seeds, wait until the seed pods change color. To confirm if they are ready, just give the pods a tap; if seeds fall out, they are ready to be gathered.

It is important to harvest your crop from healthy plants in order to obtain the best extracts. The active agents and volatile oils will be plentiful. When collecting herbs, it is best to avoid contamination of aromas by placing each cutting in a separate collection bag; this will preserve the fragrance and oil content.

Harvesting Herb Parts

Leaves and Stems Select the young fresh leaves and stems before they undergo a tough and woody transformation.

Seeds Collect the seed heads or seed pods before they become overripe. Cut them and store them in a warm, dry place to ripen.

Flowers As the flower opens and reaches its peak, cut it from the stem just below the flower head.

Berries and Fruits These are best collected when ripe but before they become overripe or subjected to injury from the birds. Pick the fruits and use immediately or preserve.

Rhizomes, Roots and Tubers Once the above-ground stems and leaves have died and the plant goes into a dormant state, collect the underground structures.

Woods and Bark Many plants have bark or wood that can be used. Never cut bark away in a circular manner from the plant as this gives it no protection from infection. Collect the bark from harvested twigs or branches, making sure to seal any cut areas left after their removal.

DRYING HERBS

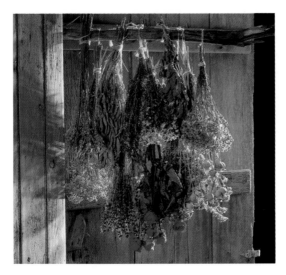

Air-drying is the most natural way for preserving herbs, and they look attractive hung upside down in bunches.

THE BEST HERBS to dry are thyme, tarragon, bay leaves and rosemary. These hold their aroma and taste for a good long time, but for most herbs there is no comparison to that of a freshly picked sprig. In general it is not wise to keep dried herbs for more than 12 months since the aroma and flavor will reduce dramatically after this period.

When drying the leaves, it is best to collect them just before the buds open to make sure that the leaves contain the highest concentrations of oils and essential agents. Herbs such as thyme and tarragon can be tied together and hung in bunches to dry. For the larger-leaf varieties of herbs, such as mint, basil and sage, pick only perfect leaves early in the day before the sun has a chance to dry out the essential oils. Once they have been picked, hang the bundles in a warm place (an airing cupboard is perfect) to dry out to a point where they are brittle enough to crumble and store in a bottle.

Once your herbs are dried, keep them in individual storage bottles that are clearly marked with the name of the herb and the date harvested. The bottles need to be clean, airtight and kept in a dry, dark place.

Air-Drying

This is the most widely used and easiest method of preserving the herbs. Simply spread them out on a dry surface or bunch them up and tie with a length of twine. The herbs should be dried within two days, otherwise the potency of aroma and effectiveness of the active agents will decline dramatically. If the leaves turn a dark brown-black and show signs of mold, then the process is too slow, and the herb has become unusable. Ideal drying conditions are 68°–73°F (20°–23°C) in a dry and fume-free environment. The traditional method of hanging the herbs in bunches will increase the efficiency of the drying method. Spread flowers and large leaves out on blotting paper and allow to dry on a wire cooling rack.

Seed heads should be hung upside down so that the seeds may fall out during the drying process and land on a piece of clean blotting paper placed underneath.

Oven-Drying

This method is not recommended for fragile leaves and flowers because heat will destroy all the active agents and oils. Oven-drying is most suitable for the larger structures, such as roots, rhizomes and tubers, which need intense drying at 122°–140°F (50°–60°C) for successful preservation. The drying process will take about three hours.

Storage Containers

Once your herbs have been dried, the containers in which they are stored will make all the difference to their shelf life. A clear glass container will allow the herbs to become bleached by light, which damages the valuable chemicals contained within the plants. Plastic containers may encourage a moist atmosphere that in turn can cause molds to grow and spoil the dried preparations. The best containers are dark glass or ceramic pots with airtight lids. These protect the contents from becoming damaged by light or air. Keeping these containers in a cool, dark place will increase the shelf life of the herbs.

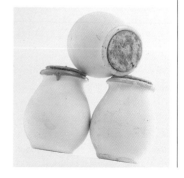

MAKING REMEDIES

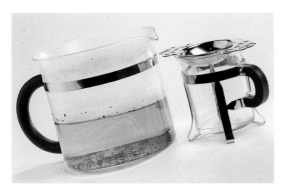

*A relaxing infusion of Chamomile (*Anthemis nobilis*)*

Infusions and Decoctions

Infusions are made by adding boiling water to the delicate parts of the herb—the flowers, leaves and seeds. An infusion is normally made from a single herb, and it should never consist of more than three herbs.

To make an infusion, try mixing 1 oz (25 g) dried herb, or double this amount for a fresh herb, with 2½ cups (600 ml/ 1 pint) boiling water. Pour the boiling water over the herbs, cover and leave to steep for 15 minutes. Strain the mixture, squeeze out the herbs to obtain the maximum amount of juice, and drink a cupful twice daily. Good herbs to experiment with include sage, mint and chamomile.

For the hardy parts of a plant—the wood, bark and stems— a decoction is used to extract the active agents from this tough material. The same quantities are used as for an infusion, but the water and herbs are brought to a boil from cold, then simmered for 20 minutes before they are strained and drunk.

Infusion and decoction preparations are best taken the day they are made, but they can be kept in the refrigerator for about 24 hours.

Tinctures

The herbs (any part can be used) are steeped for just over two weeks in an alcohol-and-water mixture. The process extracts the active agents out of the plant matter, while the alcohol content of the mixture preserves the tincture for about two years from the date of manufacture. After about two weeks, press out the mixture to obtain the final tincture. Seal in an airtight container and use as needed. It is best to make tinctures of single herbs and only combine them with other tinctures when needed. Your local pharmacy can supply you with the alcohol needed for the extraction process. Commercial tinctures use ethyl alcohol but you can make tinctures at home using vodka (37.5%). Dilute 3¼ cups (750 ml) vodka with 2½ tablespoons (37.5 ml) water and use this mixture to steep the herbs in.

Oils

The extraction of oils from plant material is a complex process. The majority of oils are extracted by steam distillation. In this method water is heated to its boiling point, and the steam is directed to a large chamber containing the herbs. As the steam passes through the bed of herbal material, vaporized water and essential oils are released. These run through a condenser to be collected as oil and floral water. Oils such as lavender, myrrh, sandalwood and cinnamon are collected in this way.

The process isolates the volatile oil from the plant material. Other substances such as tannins and bitters are excluded from collection. A redistillation at different temperatures can separate different constituents of the essential oil such as camphor, which can be broken down by further distillation into white, yellow or brown camphor. Essential oils tend to evaporate when brought into contact with the air, so it is vitally important to keep the lids on bottles of essential oils firmly closed to preserve the aroma.

When mixing oils for use in massage, it is recommended that the combination be kept simple, and no more than four oils are used together in any one remedy. It is perfectly acceptable to use a single oil, and this may actually exert a more powerful effect than if it were combined with others.

Oils in Massage Oils for use in massage have been classified according to the part of the plant from which they have been extracted. Oils derived from the flowers are termed the top notes and carry the presenting aroma that is first noticed; those from the leaves are called the middle notes and have a more therapeutic action; oils from the wood and roots are known as the base notes as they provide a "fixing" characteristic to a blend since they have a more long-lasting aroma. A formula with a balanced blend of oils, therefore, carries all of these notes.

The oil into which the essential oils are mixed is referred to as the carrier, or base, oil and is commonly grapeseed or almond oil. Others, such as wheatgerm or avocado oil, can be used, but these are normally reserved for very dry skin types because of the nutritive nature of the oil.

Oils in the Bath The addition of a few drops (about five) of essential oil to a bath can be very relaxing and therapeutic. For those with very sensitive skin, this method of use may cause irritation, and the advice of a professional aromatherapist is best sought. Try a bath with chamomile or lavender to relieve stress or insomnia or rosemary oil to help aching muscles and stiff joints.

Oils in Vaporization Making use of the evaporative properties of essential oils can be a fun and delightful way to scent a room. Placing a few drops over a piece of tissue paper draped over a radiator can generate a marvelous aroma in the

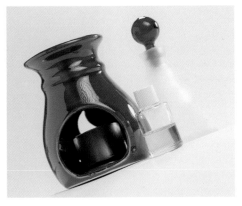

Burning a few drops of essential oil in a burner is a great way to scent a room.

room, strong enough to clear the air of unwanted cigarette smoke if needed. When taken to the sick room, essential oils can help purify the air and ease the congested breathing of the bed-bound patient. The oils may even lift his or her mood. Try vaporizing essential oils of eucalyptus or peppermint in the sick room.

To lift the mood and induce relaxation, fill a room with the fragrance of cedarwood and frankincense. This can be achieved by using an oil burner or placing a few drops around the light bulb ring used to fasten a shade to the light fitting.

Oils in Steam Inhalation

There is no better way to clear the chest and sinuses than by the traditional method of steam inhalation. Add three to five drops of peppermint, eucalyptus or thyme to a bowl of hot water, cover your head with a towel and lean over the steam. Breathe in deeply and feel the passages clear.

> **CAUTIONARY NOTE:**
> In certain sensitive asthmatic people, the oils used and the steam itself may trigger attacks during the inhalation treatment. It is strongly advised that professional guidance is followed when using this method of treatment in an asthmatic person.

Oils Taken Internally The internal use of essential oils is not recommended unless you have been given specific instructions on what oil to use and how much to take. Many oils can be extremely irritating to the stomach and may cause serious adverse reactions when taken this way.

Poultices and Compresses

The best method of making a poultice is to use the fresh leaves, stems and roots. Chop and crush the material into a paste, adding water as needed to form a good consistency. A short whiz in a blender or food processor can speed up the process. The final processed herb can be either applied directly to the skin or placed between two thin layers of gauze and bound firmly to the area.

The poultice can be bearably hot or cold, but the best method of keeping it active is to place a hot water bottle over the gauze for about 30 minutes. This can be repeated every two to three hours as needed.

A poultice made from bread can help ripen a boil and bring the infection to the surface, while one made from cabbage leaves can bring great relief to arthritic joints.

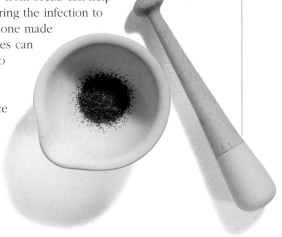

For a compress, simply soak a piece of cotton fabric or clean dish towel in a fresh herbal infusion (hot or cold), a decoction or diluted herbal tincture. Apply it directly to the affected area. When using a hot infusion, allow the compress to cool before changing it. If a cold application is used, repeat when the compress dries out. A compress is best used when healing is needed, especially when there is damage to muscles and ligaments.

Ointments and Creams

Ointments are designed to sit on the skin, especially in areas of weakness or where extra moisture is needed. They are made of oils and fats (such as petroleum jelly or paraffin wax) and contain no water. Any herbs can be used but comfrey (*Symphytum officinale*), calendula (*Calendula officinalis*) and goldenseal (*Hydrastis canadensis*) are particularly beneficial.

Once you have melted down the oil or wax of your choice using a double boiler, slowly add your chosen herbs. Continue to heat for about two hours. Remove from the heat and filter the mixture into a bowl using a piece of cheesecloth, squeezing out the mixture thoroughly. Decant the liquid quickly into clean jars and leave to solidify. Use as required.

Creams are used when the herb needs to be absorbed into the skin. Obtain some emulsifying ointment from your local pharmacy. Melt this down and add a little water and the herbs, then slowly heat the mixture for about two-and-a-half hours. Filter the mixture through a cheesecloth and squeeze out firmly. Transfer the cream to clean jars and store in a cool place. Your cream may be kept in this way for two months.

MEDICINAL USES

IT IS IMPORTANT to keep in mind that plant extracts can be very toxic as well as beneficial to health. Just because they are natural does not mean they are safe; some of the most powerful poisons are obtained from plants.

In order to make the use of herbal medicine safe and effective, you need to know how much and how often to take an extract. Just as a medicine bottle from the pharmacy tells you how much aspirin is in each tablet, so a bottle of herbal medicine should tell you how much active agent is contained in it. This not only safeguards against overdosage, but it also reassures you that you are taking a good-quality extract. Consider the label taken from an over-the-counter remedy (see box).

What does this mean? The common name is given as well as the botanical name, thus allowing for a complete understanding of the extract contained in the preparation. The dosage, given in milligrams, gives

> Korean ginseng root extract (3:1)
> (*Panax ginseng*) 100 mg
> Siberian ginseng root extract (5:1)
> (*Eleutherococcus senticosus*) 150 mg
> Standardized to contain 1% eleutheroside

the weight of root extract, but only when the extraction concentration is given (e.g. 3:1 or 5:1) do you know how strong the extract is. When the extract is expressed in the form 3:1, this means that each tablet or capsule has the same potency as three capsules of the powdered herb; 5:1 means that each capsule has the same potency as five capsules of the powdered herb. In other words, the extract has been concentrated.

When an extract has been standardized, its content is at a pharmaceutical grade and is consistent. The 1 percent eleutheroside in the example states that the dose of the active agent for that manufacturer's ginseng compound is one percent. A poor-quality ginseng will still weigh the same when powdered, but there is no law at present that requires the manufacturer to tell the customer if the extract actually contains any active agent, so it is well worth understanding how to read the labels.

With a liquid tincture, the descriptive terms change again. Tinctures are normally made at a dose of 1:5 or 1:10 concentration, meaning that one part herb is soaked in five or 10 parts liquid. In other words, they include five or 10 times the amount of solvent than herb. Tinctures are normally made by using a water-and-alcohol solvent. The herb is soaked in this solvent for hours to sometimes days before being squeezed out and bottled as a tincture.

Fluid extracts are made by soaking the herbs in solvents such as vinegar, glycol or glycerin, and then distilling off some of the liquid using vacuum distillation or countercurrent distillation, both of which achieve the final 1:1 concentration without using heat. This leaves one part herb to one part solvent. Fluid extracts are, therefore, five to 10 times stronger than tinctures.

Solid extracts are generally made by thin-layer evaporation methods, in which the solvent is completely removed, leaving behind the dry, solid plant material. This can be finely powdered and used to fill capsules. The powdered extract can be reconstituted by adding back the water or alcohol. Probably one of the greatest improvements that modern science has been able to offer herbal medicine is the ability to produce pure, safe and standardized methods of extraction. This has aided the effective use of herbal remedies as well as the research into the plant constituents. The ability to offer the herbal user a standardized extract allows a universal understanding of the dose taken regardless of the crop quality or method of extraction.

Standardized Extracts

Since the beginning of time, people have used herbs to promote health and well-being. To make the best possible use of herbal extracts, pure standardized extracts (PSE) have been developed to ensure the highest level of quality and consistency. To obtain a PSE, concentrate the herb by mixing the crude plant with an appropriate amount of alcohol and water. The alcohol and water is then either partially or completely removed to produce a liquid, soft or solid extract. Making an herbal extract is rather like refining pure gold from crude ore.

These modern laboratory methods preserve the beneficial botanical compounds. These extracts are normally available in capsules as a dry or powdered form because this offers the greatest stability to the final extract.

The PSE is not a method of isolating chemicals. All PSE formulas contain the same chemicals found in the crude plant including essential oils, flavonoids, alkaloids, glucosides and saponins. It is important not only to have these compounds present, but also to have them in the proper ratio.

Importance of Standardization

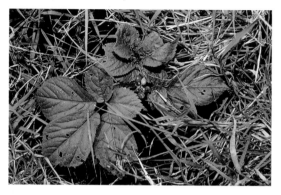

*Korean ginseng (*Panax ginseng*) is used to improve stamina.*

Herbs can vary tremendously in chemical composition and quality depending on where they are grown, soil factors and how and when they are harvested. A nonstandardized herbal remedy cannot, therefore, guarantee any consistency.

To consider an example, Korean ginseng (*Panax ginseng*) has been featured in a number of studies. Independent research and published studies have clearly shown a tremendous variation in the content of the active agent, called ginsenoside, in commercial preparations. Most contained only trace amounts of ginsenoside, while some contained none at all! To solve this problem, manufacturers of herbal preparations needed to guarantee the level of these compounds. The method of preparation and extraction needed to do this is the PSE process. This gives manufacturers the ability to state, for example, "*Panax ginseng* standardized to contain 17 percent ginsenosides." This method allows the user of herbal preparations to be aware of the exact strength of the preparation he is taking and to be reassured that it will be consistent.

The Phytosome® Method

This method is probably the most advanced way of preparing an herbal extract for human use. Phytosomes are created when herbal molecules are bound to phosphatidylcholine, a natural component of lecithin, which is found throughout the body in our cell membranes. The Phytosome method allows a water-soluble herbal extract to be surrounded by a coat that makes it readily absorbable across a cell membrane. The cells will actively take up this Phytosome complex from the circulation. Herbal extracts normally find their way into cells by a process of passive diffusion. This process intensifies the herbal compounds by improving their absorption and increasing their biological availability. Some herbal compounds are not very bioavailable, and very large doses are needed for an effect to be noticed. The Phytosome process has revolutionized the use of such herbs.

Medicine Cabinet Staples

There are a number of essential herbs that are best kept as tinctures or ready-made tablets or capsules so that they are always ready for instant use. Tinctures of echinacea (*Echinacea purpura*) and valerian (*Valeriana officinalis*) are always good to have in store, as well as preparations of licorice (*Glycyrrhiza glabra*), Korean ginseng (*Panax ginseng*) and cranberry (*Vaccinium macrocarpon*).

The choice and variations of herbs to keep in the medicine cabinet are almost limitless and are dependent on you and your family's needs.

Basic Medicinal Herbs

Aloe vera (*Alo barbadensis*)
Chamomile (*Anthemis nobilis*)
Cranberry (*Vaccinium macrocarpon*)
Echinacea (*Echinacea purpura*)
Feverfew (*Tanacetum parthenium*)
Garlic (*Allium sativum*)
Ginger (*Zingiber officinalis*)
Ginseng (*Panax ginseng*)
Licorice (*Glycyrrhiza glabra*)
Valerian (*Valeriana officinalis*)

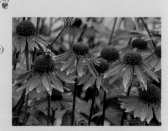

*Echinacea (*Echinacea purpura*) stimulates the immune system.*

COSMETIC USES

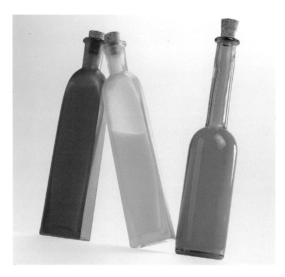

*Making your own cosmetic preparations is rewarding
as only natural ingredients are used.*

PLANT EXTRACTS HAVE been used in body painting since
the time of the ancient Egyptians. Woad (a blue dye
obtained from *Isatis tinctoria*) was used by the ancient Britons
to paint their bodies much in a way similar Native Americans
used plant dyes and oils.

Flower Water

Many plants can be used fresh or dried. Plants with aromatic
leaves are most effective at the end of summer, but they are
considered to be freshest at the start of summer. These plants
can be dried and, when stored correctly, can be used
throughout the year. For best results the plants need to be
dried just after picking in order to preserve the aromatic oils.

After rinsing the plant in cold water and removing all the
dead material, place in a clean pan that is big enough to hold
two handfuls of plants. Add enough water to cover the
material. Then cook the plants over low heat to release the
aromatic oils. In general, cook the plants 15–20 minutes. After
cooking, strain the mixture, decant into small storage jars and
transfer to a cold place to keep the extracts fresh.

Cleansing Milk

1 cup (250 ml/8 fl oz) buttermilk
2 tablespoons chamomile flowers
2 tablespoons elder blossom
2 tablespoons lime blossom

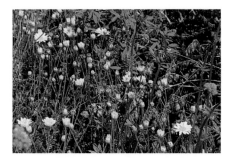

Chamomile (Anthemis nobilis)

Place all the ingredients in a pan and simmer for 30 minutes; do not allow the mixture to boil. After simmering, leave the mixture to cool for just over two hours before straining and decanting into a storage bottle. Store in the refrigerator and use within a week of making. Use the cleansing milk before the herbal toning lotion.

Toning Lotion

Mix together equal parts of flower waters (rose, lavender, elderflower and orange), combine and mix well. Take 2 tablespoons of the mixture and add it to 2 tablespoons lemon juice and 2 tablespoons witch hazel. For a soothing effect, add a few drops of essential oil (lavender, geranium or rose), and mix the ingredients together well. Store the lotion in a cool place, and apply morning and evening to restore the skin's natural texture and cleanse the pores.

Astringent

Infuse a good handful of lime blossom or meadowsweet flowers, allow to cool, and then strain. Mix 1¼ cups (300 ml/ ½ pint) boiling water with 1 teaspoon witch hazel. Then combine the flower water with the witch hazel mixture.

Witch hazel has the ability to soothe and soften skin while acting as a deep cleansing agent. Use this formulation morning and evening.

HOME USES

HERBS AND AROMATIC plants have been used in the home for centuries. Potpourri and incense balls were widely used in medieval times for freshening the air. The ancient Egyptians were also known to use combinations of aromatic herbs in rooms for decorative and medicinal purposes.

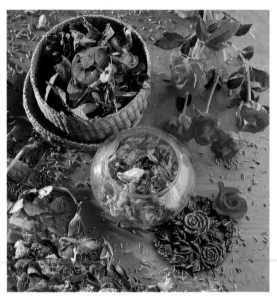

*Lavender (*Lavandula officinalis*) is one of the few flowers to retain their aroma after drying and is ideal for potpourris.*

Potpourri

Making a potpourri can introduce a unique aromatic characteristic to your living room or bedroom. A potpourri comprises four component parts—flowers, leaves, spices and a fixative (called the base note in aromatherapy). The fixative is needed to keep the potpourri together. The aromatic substance chosen releases its scent slowly, giving a long-lasting aroma to the mixture.

The advantage of making your own potpourri, rather than buying it, is that you can choose the combination that will suit your taste exactly. Select the ingredients for your potpourri from the following suggestions.

FLOWERS
- Elder
- Honeysuckle
- Lavender
- Lily-of-the-valley
- Lime blossom
- Narcissus
- Orange blossom
- Rose
- Sweet rocket

AROMATIC LEAVES
- Basil
- Bay
- Bergamot
- Lemon balm
- Lemon verbena
- Rosemary
- Sage
- Sweet marjoram
- Tarragon

- Thyme
- Woodruff

SPICES
- Allspice
- Aniseed
- Cardamom
- Cloves
- Coriander
- Dill seeds
- Ginger
- Nutmeg
- Star anise
- Vanilla beans

BASE-NOTE FRAGRANCES
- Frankincense
- Myrrh
- Sandalwood
- Sweet flag root

Potpourri must be aged before using. Place in a sealed container and leave in a warm, dry place for four to six weeks.

Drying the Flowers The ideal drying temperature is about 75°F (24°C). The flowers need to be spread out evenly, without overlapping, on gauze or newspaper. They will need to be turned every day. For an effective drying process, the smaller petals need to be dried for up to seven days, while larger, thicker petals may take up to three weeks to be fully dried. Flowers such as lavender and chamomile can be dried on the stem and are best tied in bunches and hung upside down for drying.

Spicy Spring Potpourri

Flowers
3 cups rose petals

2 cups lavender

1 cup cloves

Leaves
¼ cup rosemary

½ cup bergamot

¼ cup bay leaves

½ cup southernwood

Colored Flowers
¼ cup calendula

½ cup forget-me-not

Spices
½ tablespoon ground cloves

1 tablespoon allspice

Base-note Fixative Oil
5 tablespoons sandalwood oil

CULINARY USES

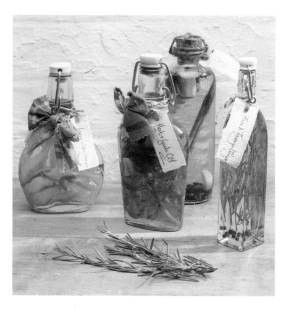

Aromatic oils are useful for adding flavor to any salad dressing. All oils should be kept in a cool, dark place.

W HEN USED IN cooking, the tender aromatic plant tips tend to be classified as herbs, while the dried aromatic extracts of the plants' barks, flower buds, fruits, seeds and roots are known collectively as spices. The term "condiments" refers to spices that are added to the food at the table after cooking.

Many composite spices and herbs are also available. Apple spice is a mixture of cinnamon, nutmeg and sugar as well as other aromatic spices. Pumpkin spice is made by mixing cinnamon, ginger, nutmeg and cloves. For savory foods, a good meat tenderizer can be made from salt and papain (from the pawpaw fruit). On the barbecue, try using a mixture of Indian and Italian herbs to create a special flavor.

There is also an interesting variety of composite condiments available. These often contain sea salt and a mixture of up to 16 different herbs such as bell peppers, garlic, onion and many others. The herbal salt combination Herbamare (produced by Bioforce) is prepared from organically grown herbs that have been allowed to steep with sea salt for six to eight weeks before the moisture is removed using a special vacuum method at low temperature. This method of manufacture preserves the aroma and flavor of the herbal ingredients. Herbamare, therefore, contains nutrients and natural plant-based iodine. This salt combination is based in celery leaves, leeks, celery root, watercress, onions, chives, parsley, lovage, basil, marjoram, rosemary, thyme and kelp. A similar method of production is used in the manufacture of a more spicy version, Trocomare, which also contains horseradish and red bell pepper.

It is important to remember that the art of flavoring in cooking is to use just enough to enhance the dish, not to overpower the final result with the flavor of the herbs. As a rule, ground spices lose their flavor quickly and are not suitable for dishes that require long cooking times. For stews or soups, add them within the last 20 minutes before serving.

In most cases, use at least twice the amount of fresh herb to give the same intensity of flavor as its dried equivalent, but remember that the flavor quality of the fresh herb cannot be compared to the dried. Different herbs and spices have an affinity with different foods, which makes cooking an exciting and enjoyable activity.

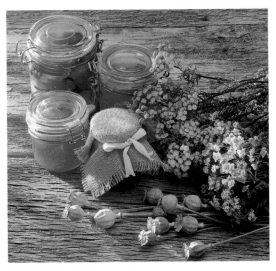

Herbs can be added to preserves to enhance the flavor.
A single or a mixture of herbs makes delicious combinations.

Herbs for Cooking

Garlic (*Allium sativum*) Garlic tends to be more pungent than onion. Do not use a wooden board for chopping or crushing it because the wood will become saturated with the aromatic oils. Use garlic in soups, fish dishes, roast lamb, meat stews, poultry dishes and pasta. Vegetables are especially good when prepared using garlic. Try it with tomatoes, green bell peppers, artichokes, eggplant and spinach. Vinaigrette dressing would not be the same without a good dash of garlic. Also try using garlic in marinades and mixed with butter for oven-baked garlic bread.

Chives (*Allium schoenoprasum*) Chives give a mild onion flavor that is best released by snipping the leaves and adding them to the dish immediately before the oils evaporate. Try adding chives to vegetables of all kinds, fish, salads, baked potatoes, omelets and egg dishes. As a garnish, chives are irreplaceable as a source of color. Chives mix well with chopped parsley. Use the flowers to garnish soups and savory dishes.

Dill (*Anethum graveolens*) Dill has a slight anise flavor. Use the chopped leaves in salads, vegetable dishes (they are especially good with large zucchini, tomatoes, beets and cabbage) and egg dishes. Use a sprig and the leaves as garnishes for fish. The seeds may be used in fish dishes, grilled lamb and pork, stews, sauerkraut and cabbage. Dill is also a good addition to cheese dishes.

Angelica (*Angelica archangelica*) Angelica has a penetrating flavor. Care is needed since some may find the taste overpowering. The stems are crystalized and used to decorate cakes and desserts. Try using the leaves and roots for stewing with fruit to give an alternative sweetness to sugar. Chopped angelica may be used in salads, hot wine and fruit drinks.

Horseradish (*Armoracia rusticana*) Horseradish gives off a hot, strong and pungent aroma rather like mustard. When shredded, the root can be used as a sauce, mixed with cream and vinegar. Add to shellfish and smoked fish dishes. As the classic accompaniment to roast beef, it is said to help digestion. Other foods that work well with horseradish include poultry, beets and tomatoes.

Caraway Seeds (*Carum carvi*) Caraway seeds have a licorice flavor that's stronger than anise. The whole seeds are used in dumplings for soups and stews, goulash and vegetable dishes, especially red and white cabbage, cauliflower, beets, turnips and potatoes. Try adding the seeds to a rye bread mix or just to a standard bread mix for a special flavor and aroma. Grind the seeds when adding caraway to stews and vegetables such as zucchini, beans, cabbage, tomatoes and potato salad.

Cilantro (*Coriandrum sativum*) Cilantro is a versatile herb and the leaves and green coriander seeds have a very pungent aroma. Use a small handful of young chopped leaves in soups, beef stews, poultry dishes, salads, vegetables and even desserts. Try adding the leaves and green seeds to curries.

Turmeric (*Curcuma longa*) Turmeric is unmistakable with its distinctive color and delicate aroma. It is used ground in fish and shellfish dishes, curries, stews and in rice and vegetable dishes. Try adding a little turmeric to homemade relish and chutneys.

Fennel (*Foeniculum vulgare*) Fennel has a more concentrated flavor than dill and has the similar anise taste. It goes very well with fish, particularly the oily types. Try grilling the fish over sprigs of dried fennel. Otherwise, use it in exactly the same way as dill. The seeds can be used in a fish bouillon or try adding them to bread mixes.

Hyssop (*Hyssopus officinalis*) Hyssop is slightly bitter with a hint of mint. The tender young leaves can be used in soups and with oily fish. Stews, salads, stuffing mixes and fruit cocktails also benefit from the addition of hyssop. Cranberries, peaches and apricots are delicious with hyssop.

Juniper Berries (*Juniperus communis*) Juniper berries are generally used dried. They can be lightly crushed to release their strong bittersweet flavor. Try adding a small handful of berries to rice dishes, sauces, marinades and relish, or use them with game meats, pork and as a delicious ingredient in stuffing mix.

Bay Leaves (*Laurus nobilis*) Bay leaves should be added at the start of cooking. They deliver a strong spicy flavor to soups and stews. Bay can be added to all meat dishes. For sweet dishes, try adding it to milk desserts and custards.

Bay leaves form an essential part of a bouquet garni. To make, take one bay leaf, three or four sprigs of parsley, including stalks, and a sprig of thyme, and wrap in a small piece of cheesecloth, and tie tightly. You can add other herbs to taste.

Peppermint (*Mentha piperita*) Peppermint leaves are great added to a salad or desserts and jellies.

Basil (*Ocimum basilicum*) Basil gives a peppery flavor to a dish. The leaves, torn not chopped, may be added to soups, fish, egg and game dishes. Try basil mixed with rice, vegetables or pasta during cooking. Finely grind and use as part of a vinaigrette dressing for salads.

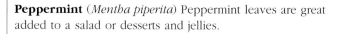

Sweet Marjoram (*Origanum majorana*) Sweet marjoram has a sweet and spicy flavor and is very versatile in cooking. The leaves can be chopped and added to soups or meat dishes, poultry and vegetables. Potatoes, carrots, cabbage and celery are especially good mixed with a little marjoram. Try adding it to cheese, egg and fish dishes. Oregano (*Origanum vulgare*) belongs to the same family as sweet marjoram but has a stronger flavor. Use chopped leaves in salads and pasta dishes.

Parsley (*Petroselinum crispum*) Parsley can be considered one of the most versatile herbs with its own distinctive flavor. The stalks have a stronger flavor than the leaves, so in stews, stocks and marinades it is best to use the stalks. For a bouquet garni, try adding the whole sprig. For soups, fish dishes, meat and poultry, use the freshly chopped leaves. As a garnish, parsley adds color and texture to any dish.

Rosemary (*Rosmarinus officinalis*) Rosemary can overpower a dish because it is a very strong and aromatic herb. Use whole sprigs under roast lamb or placed inside a chicken. The chopped leaves are suitable for soups, fish dishes, bacon, ham and any meat or game stew. Rosemary combines well with large zucchini, peas, bell peppers, potatoes and bread mixes.

Sage (*Salvia officinalis*) Sage has a strong and distinctive flavor. It is slightly bitter and goes well with fatty foods probably because it stimulates the flow of bile that aids fat digestion. The chopped leaves go very well with pork, duck and sausages. With vegetables, sage combines well with tomatoes, bell peppers, dried beans, eggplant and onions. In a stuffing, sage is a vital ingredient.

Cloves (*Syzygium aromaticum*) Cloves have an unmistakable sharp and spicy flavor. The whole clove can be stuck into an onion and added to soups or stews to produce an aromatic flavor to the finished dish. Try studding a ham or beef with cloves before cooking. Use the ground spice in meat dishes and curries with vegetables. Cloves go very well with beets, sweet potatoes and Belgian endive. Baked fruit and fruit pie fillings lend themselves to spicing up with a few cloves. Use ground cloves in pumpkin pie. Mulled wine and ale should never be without cloves.

Thyme (*Thymus vulgaris*) Thyme has a distinctive, strong flavor. A sprig of thyme is a must in a bouquet garni, stocks and marinades. The chopped leaves may be added to soups, fish and shellfish dishes, meat and poultry. It is a very versatile herb, combining well with beets, mushrooms, pasta, rice, tomatoes, beans and bread mix.

Fenugreek (*Trigonella foenum-graecum*) Fenugreek has a background flavor of bitterness. Use it ground in vegetable and bean soups, curries, meat stews and homemade chutneys.

Ginger (*Zingiber officinale*) Ginger, when fresh, gives off a fabulous aroma. The hot, strong characteristics of this spice make it a good accompaniment to Chinese and Indian food. Use the whole dried root in relish and chutneys. When ground it can be scattered over melon or grapefruit and added to soups, vegetable dishes and cake mixes.

Culinary Cupboard Staples

If you like to experiment in the kitchen and you have advanced cooking skills, a wide range of herbs is essential. If, however, your culinary expertise is limited, then choose a basic range of herbs. It might be wise to start with just parsley, sage, bay, peppermint, garlic, cilantro, oregano, cloves and ginger; then, as your confidence increases, you could add to the selection you keep in stock.

Basic Culinary Herbs

Basil	Parsley
Bay	Peppermint
Cilantro	Rosemary
Fennel	Sage
Garlic	Sweet Marjoram
Ginger	Tarragon
Oregano	Thyme

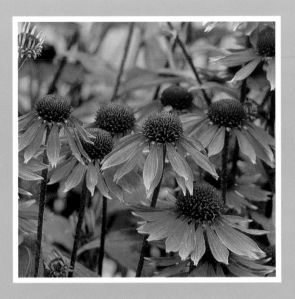

THE HERB
DIRECTORY

HERB LIST
BY COMMON NAME

Agrimony	*Agrimonia eupatoria*	51
Alfalfa	*Medicago sativa*	108
Aloe vera	*Alo barbadensis*	56
American cranesbill	*Geranium maculatum*	94
Angelica	*Angelica archangelica*	59
Arnica	*Arnica montana*	67
Artichoke	*Cynara scolymus*	84
Astragalus	*Astragalus membranaceus*	70
Basil	*Ocimum basilicum*	111
Bilberry	*Vaccinium myrtillus*	150
Black cohosh	*Cimicifuga racemosa*	79
Blackthorn	*Prunus spinosa*	124
Borage	*Borago officinalis*	72
Burdock	*Arctium lappa*	64
Butcher's broom	*Ruscus aculeatus*	128
Calendula	*Calendula officinalis*	73
Californian poppy	*Eschscholzia californica*	88
Caraway	*Carum carvi*	76
Cayenne	*Capsicum frutescens*	74
Celery	*Apium graveolens*	63
Centaury	*Centaurium erythraea*	77
Chives	*Allium schoenoprasum*	55
Cilantro	*Coriandrum sativum*	81
Clary	*Salvia sclarea*	132
Cloves	*Syzygium aromaticum*	139
Coltsfoot	*Tussilago farfara*	145
Comfrey	*Symphytum officinale*	137
Crampbark	*Viburnum opulus*	154
Cranberry	*Vaccinium macrocarpon*	148
Dandelion	*Taraxacum officinale*	142
Devil's claw	*Martynia annua*	107
Dill	*Anethum graveolens*	58
Echinacea	*Echinacea purpura*	85
Elder	*Sambucus nigra*	133
Eucalyptus	*Eucalyptus globulus*	89
Evening primrose	*Oenothera biennis*	112
Eyebright	*Euphrasis officinalis*	91
Fennel	*Foeniculum vulgare*	92
Fenugreek	*Trigonella foenum-graecum*	144
Feverfew	*Tanacetum parthenium*	140
Garlic	*Allium sativum*	53
Ginger	*Zingiber officinale*	156
Ginkgo	*Ginkgo biloba*	95
Ginseng	*Panax ginseng*	117
Ginseng (Siberian)	*Eleutherococcus senticosus*	86
Goldenseal	*Hydrastis canadensis*	98

YARROW

Achillea millefolium

THE LATIN NAME for this plant is believed to come from the Greek hero Achilles. It is said that he used it to heal his soldiers' wounds during the Trojan War.

Taken internally, this herb is used to stimulate the circulatory system and help reduce blood pressure. It has a diaphoretic action, so it is helpful in reducing fevers brought about by colds and flu. Yarrow has antiseptic and anti-inflammatory properties, so it is used to control excessive bleeding and helps reduce diarrhea and dysentery. This herb can be used to relieve indigestion, flatulence and dyspepsia.

Externally, yarrow is used to help heal minor wounds and for cleansing and toning the skin.

PARTS USED
❦ *Leaves and flowers*

DOSAGE
❦ *As a tea, add about 2 teaspoons (5–10 ml) of herbs to 2½ cups (600 ml/1 pint) of boiling water and infuse for 5 minutes.*
❦ *For external application, use as a poultice for minor cuts and scrapes.*

POTENTIAL BENEFITS
❦ *Stimulates the circulatory system*
❦ *Helps reduce blood pressure*
❦ *Helps to reduce fevers*

❦ *Has antiseptic properties*
❦ *Has anti-inflammatory properties*
❦ *Can reduce diarrhea*
❦ *Can relieve indigestion*

COSMETIC USES
❦ *Flowers can be used in creams and lotions to cleanse the skin. Yarrow can also be used in skin tonics as an astringent for oily skin.*

CULINARY USES
❦ *The fresh young leaves are used in salads.*

WARNING: Do not use yarrow for long periods as it may cause skin irritation. Avoid during pregnancy.

SWEET FLAG

Acorus calamus

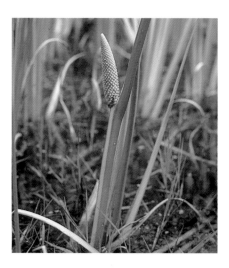

This herb has both medicinal and culinary uses. Candy made from this plant is produced by crystalizing tender slices of the roots (rhizomes). The roots contain volatile oils that have profound antibiotic actions. Taken internally, sweet flag can be very useful in the stimulation of digestion and as a remedy for bronchitis and sinus congestion. An external application can be used to relieve rheumatic joint and muscle pains. It is also a carminative agent and can reduce muscular spasms that are associated with nerve pains.

PARTS USED
❦ *Roots, rhizomes and oil extract*

DOSAGE
❦ *As a liquid tincture, take 20 drops twice daily before eating.*
❦ *For external application, use as a compress for joint and muscle pain.*

POTENTIAL BENEFITS
❦ *Helps bronchitis*
❦ *Reduces sinus congestion*
❦ *Stimulates digestion*
❦ *Eases joint and muscle pains*
❦ *May help in neuralgia*

CULINARY USES
❦ *Used to make candy*

HORSE CHESTNUT

Aesculus hippocastanum

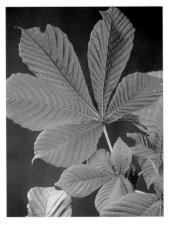

THE LEAVES OF this tree leave a horseshoe-shaped scar behind on the twig as they fall off, but it is named horse chestnut because the fruits were used as fodder for cattle and horses.

Herbal medicine has found a number of applications for this herb. When taken internally, it has a mild diuretic activity and can exert an anti-inflammatory action. This herb can improve the flow and exchange of tissue fluids in the body and can reduce the swellings associated with poor circulation. Therefore, the congestion that occurs in cases of varicose veins can be relieved by regular use of an extract of horse chestnut. Its value in circulatory problems can be seen by the benefit reported by those who have suffered a stroke or suffer from erythema or other conditions associated with poor circulation—it promotes the flow of oxygenated blood to every area of the body.

PARTS USED
- *Bark and seeds*

DOSAGE
- *As a liquid tincture, take 15–20 drops twice daily.*
- *For external application, apply as a cream directly to varicose veins as needed.*

POTENTIAL BENEFITS
- *Acts as a mild diuretic*
- *Regulates circulation*
- *Reduces tissue inflammation*
- *Eases varicose vein symptoms*
- *Promotes flow of oxygenated blood to all areas of the body*

COSMETIC USES
- *May be used in a lotion to improve the skin's circulation.*

AGRIMONY

Agrimonia eupatoria

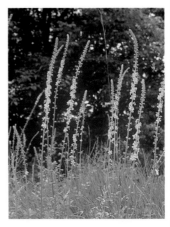

During Anglo-Saxon times, agrimony was used externally as a wound-healing agent. This use was practiced by the French during the fifteenth century, when they applied the herb after gunshot injuries. The agents responsible for the medicinal actions have been identified as astringents. These substances have the ability to close wounds and control the flow of blood.

Other medicinal functions of this plant rely on the bitter principles present in the extracts. Bitters can cause the gallbladder to contract and release its stored bile as well as stimulate the flow of digestive juices. Agrimony can reduce the inflammation of the stomach lining that often results from food allergies. Used externally, this herb can also help relieve symptoms of eczema.

PARTS USED
❦ *Whole plant*

DOSAGE
❦ *As a liquid tincture, take 20 drops twice daily before eating.*
❦ *For external application, use as a compress for eczema.*

POTENTIAL BENEFITS
❦ *Controls bleeding wounds when applied as a compress*
❦ *Assists liver function and digestion*
❦ *Helps in some cases of food allergy*
❦ *Helps reduce skin irritations from eczema*

COSMETIC USES
❦ *The leaves can be used in a facial wash to improve the skin's complexion.*

LADY'S MANTLE

Alchemilla vulgaris

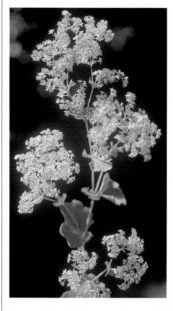

THE LEAVES OF Lady's mantle were considered to hold special magical powers once, so much so that the translation of its botanical name, *Alchemilla*, means "little magical one."

It has been used for many feminine problems and was thought to restore a lady's beauty. In the treatment of menopausal disorders, the astringent and anti-inflammatory properties help control irregular bleeding, an effect that prompted its use for menstrual problems in younger women. Taken internally, lady's mantle can help regulate excessive or irregular menstrual bleeding and can also be used as a treatment for diarrhea. Applied externally, its properties make it very useful for the treatment of vaginal discharge.

PARTS USED
❧ Whole plant

DOSAGE
❧ *As a liquid tincture, take 20 drops twice daily.*
❧ *As a douche, infuse 1 tablespoon (15 ml) dried powder, strain and apply in the morning and evening.*

POTENTIAL BENEFITS
❧ *Controls excessive bleeding*
❧ *Regulates menstrual bleeding*
❧ *Aids in vaginal infections*
❧ *Relieves diarrhea*

COSMETIC USES
❧ *The leaves can be used in a lotion as an astringent to help oily skin.*

GARLIC

Allium sativum

IT SEEMS THAT not a day passes without some new benefit of garlic being discovered. The ancient Egyptians actually worshipped the herb and fed it to their slaves to keep them fit and well.

Taken internally, garlic's volatile oils keep the lungs clear of infections. The treatment of pneumonia, bronchitis and asthma should be followed up by a preventive dose of garlic daily.

The risk of heart disease due to cholesterol deposits can be reduced by regular doses of garlic. It has been shown that the "bad" cholesterol (low-density lipoproteins [LDL]) is reduced, while the "good" cholesterol (high-density lipoprotein [HDL]) is increased after garlic is ingested. At the same time the stickiness of the bloods platelets (small fragments that cause a clot to form) is dramatically reduced.

Garlic has a powerful antimicrobial action and can be applied directly to infected areas. Fungal infections, often difficult to control, can be reduced by a garlic application.

New research is suggesting that garlic contains anticancer substances, but this is still a new area of study.

The aromatic oils contained in garlic give it many of its health-promoting actions. Whenever possible, deodorized garlic preparations should not be used.

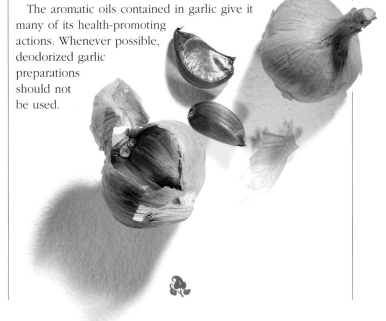

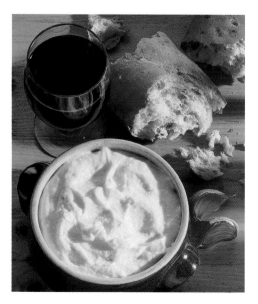

Aioli is a classic French dish and originated in Provence where it is called "beurre de Provence."

PARTS USED
🌿 Bulb

DOSAGE
🌿 Take 2 or 3 garlic capsules daily with a meal.
🌿 As a liquid tincture, take 1 or 2 teaspoons (5–10 ml) daily.
🌿 For external application, crush and apply a paste topically to the affected area.

POTENTIAL BENEFITS
🌿 Protects against heart disease
🌿 Lowers LDL cholesterol
🌿 Can reduce blood pressure
🌿 Exhibits antimicrobial activity
🌿 Kills fungi
🌿 Clears chest infections
🌿 May have cancer-protective action
🌿 Protects against blood clots

CULINARY USES
🌿 Garlic enhances the flavors of most foods. Whole, roasted garlic bulbs are sweet and mild. The dressing Aioli is made out of puréed garlic using 6–12 garlic cloves and a pinch of salt.

WARNING: When applying topically as a paste, do not tape in place because the oils can cause skin burns with chronic exposure. Eating more than five cloves at a sitting may cause a stomach upset.

CHIVES

Allium schoenoprasum

A MEMBER OF the lily family first discovered more than 5,000 years ago in China, this common herb can now be found in every food store.

Chives are high in vitamin C and iron. For this reason they are considered to be a highly nutritious food and excellent for building up the blood. Chives also have a mild stimulant effect on the appetite and can aid digestion.

PARTS USED
❦ *Leaves*

DOSAGE
❦ *Eat a large sprig of the whole herb daily.*

POTENTIAL BENEFITS
❦ *Restores blood iron levels and combats anemia*
❦ *Stimulates appetite and aids digestion*

CULINARY USES
❦ *Used in salads, soups and omelets, where onions would be too strong, and also as a garnish and in dressings. To make a chive and lemon vinaigrette, put one garlic clove and a pinch of salt in a bowl and crush together. Add the finely grated rind of one lemon, 4 tablespoons (60 ml) of lemon juice and 1½ teaspoons (7.5 ml) of mustard and stir until smooth. Slowly pour in 4*

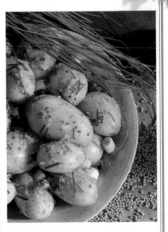

tablespoons (60 ml) of olive oil, whisking constantly until well emulsified. Add 2 teaspoons (10 ml) of chives and season with pepper. This is delicious over potatoes.

ALOE VERA
Alo barbadensis

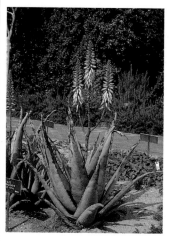

ALOE VERA IS an ancient remedy. The body of Jesus was wrapped in linen impregnated with aloe vera and myrrh.

Contained within the leaf is a special gel that is used in cosmetics as a natural skin moisturizer. A topical application of the juice can help with minor skin burns, sunburn, insect bites and sometimes with eczema.

The juice is taken internally for digestive disorders and inflammation of the stomach. The juice can be either commercially prepared or extracted from the leaves by scraping it out with the blunt side of a knife. Other benefits have been attributed to aloe vera, such as its ability to act as a natural laxative as well as an appetite stimulant.

PARTS USED
* *Leaves that contain the sap*

DOSAGE
* *Take 1 tablespoon (15 ml) juice twice daily.*
* *For external application, use as a cream or lotion on the skin as required.*

POTENTIAL BENEFITS
* *Keeps skin supple*
* *Helps speed wound healing*
* *Reduces inflammation of stomach*
* *Acts as a laxative*
* *Heals sunburn*

COSMETIC USES
* *Can be made into lotions and creams for soothing irritated and inflamed skin.*

WARNING: Internal use not advised during pregnancy. Always seek medical attention for serious burns.

MARSHMALLOW

Althaea officinalis

USED BY THE ancient Greeks in the ninth century B.C., marshmallow has been a favorite herb for the treatment of colds and chest infections including sore throats and coughs. Its soothing action can be helpful to inflammations of the stomach and lower intestine, especially in conditions such as colitis. Ulcerations of the stomach are eased with the use of marshmallow, which can make a very effective antiulcer remedy when combined with licorice. Conditions of the respiratory tract, such as asthma and bronchitis, have been reported to respond well to this herb. The peeled and washed root can be given to children to chew on as a teething aid. Used externally, marshmallow can also help heal boils and abscesses.

PARTS USED
❦ *Leaves and roots*

DOSAGE
❦ *Take 2 or 3 tablets (100 mg) of dried extract after meals.*
❦ *For external application, use as a poultice for abscesses and boils.*

POTENTIAL BENEFITS
❦ *Soothes stomach inflammation*
❦ *Helps heal stomach and skin ulcers*
❦ *Soothes colitis*
❦ *Helps speed recovery from chest infections*
❦ *Helps relieve asthma and bronchitis symptoms*
❦ *Acts as a teething aid for children*

DILL

Anethum graveolens

D ILL IS A popular culinary herb, and it has been used medicinally by doctors since ancient Egyptian and Roman times. The word "dill" comes from the Saxon word "dilla," which means to lull or soothe.

Taken internally, this herb can relieve an upset stomach and nausea. It has an antispasmodic action that helps to reduce flatulence, stimulate the appetite and aid digestion. In babies, dill can be taken to help reduce colic.

The seeds can act as a sedative, and chewing them can sweeten the breath. Dill can also stimulate the flow of breast milk in nursing mothers.

Used externally, dill is useful for soothing muscular tension. It can also be used to strengthen fingernails.

PARTS USED
❦ *Leaves and seeds*

DOSAGE
❦ *As dill water, put 2 pinches of dill seeds in 1 cup (250 ml/8 fl oz) of water and bring to a boil. As the water changes color, keep boiling for 1 minute. Strain and cool before drinking. Keep it in the refrigerator.*

❦ *As a tea, add 2 teaspoons (10 ml) of crushed seeds to 1 cup (250 ml/8 fl oz) of boiling water and let stand for 5 minutes. To reduce flatulence, drink 1 cup before eating.*

❦ *For external application, use as a compress, for muscular tension.*

❦ *For external application, use as an infusion of dill seeds to strengthen nails.*

POTENTIAL BENEFITS
❦ *Relieves nausea*
❦ *Aids digestion*
❦ *Helps reduce colic*
❦ *Stimulates the flow of breast milk in nursing mothers*
❦ *Soothes muscular tension*
❦ *Strengthens fingernails*

CULINARY USES
❦ *Popular in many dishes. Fresh leaves can be used in salads, poultry and fish dishes. Dill pickles are also popular.*

ANGELICA

Angelica archangelica

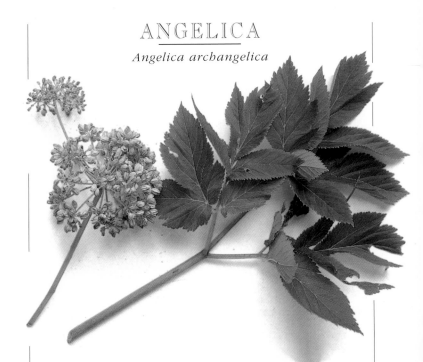

LEGEND SAYS THAT angelica was a cure for plague, which has secured it a place in traditional herbal medicine as a protector against evil.

Angelica appears to have a beneficial effect on the circulation of blood and body fluids. For the treatment of menstrual cramps and fluid retention, there can be no better herb to take than angelica. The medicinal effect that angelica exerts on the body has offered those suffering from rheumatism and arthritis a noticeable easing of symptoms. This effect may be a result of the removal of inflammatory chemicals accumulated in the tissues. Angelica is also useful in relieving symptoms of cystitis.

As a remedy for stomach upsets, gastric ulcers and migraines, angelica can be combined with chamomile (*Anthemis nobilis*). For an effective remedy against bronchitis and congestion of the lungs, angelica can be combined with yarrow (*Achillea millefolium*). An infusion can act as an expectorant in cases of colds and flu.

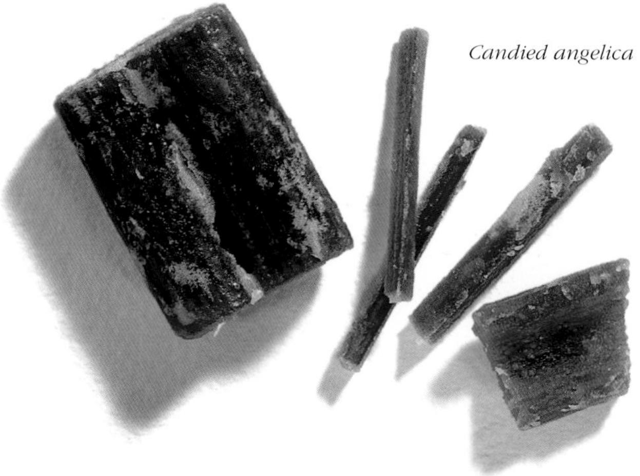

Candied angelica

PARTS USED

❦ *Leaves, seeds, stems and roots*

DOSAGE

❦ *As a liquid tincture, take 20 drops two or three times a day or 200 mg of dried herb daily.*

❦ *As an infusion add 1 tablespoon (15 ml) of dried herb to 2¼ cups (500 ml/ 18 fl oz) of boiling water.*

POTENTIAL BENEFITS

❦ *Eases symptoms of rheumatism and arthritis*

❦ *Soothes an upset stomach*

❦ *Acts as an antispasmodic to soothe menstrual cramps*

❦ *Relieves symptoms of cystitis*

❦ *Acts as an expectorant for chest infections*

CULINARY USES

❦ *Angelica leaves will give a salad a lively and aromatic flavor. The best-known application for angelica is its candied form used for cake decoration. This is not difficult to make at home. After collecting angelica stems, place them in boiling water until they are tender enough to remove the outer skins. Return the peeled stems to the pan and bring to a boil again. Cool the stems and add an equal weight of sugar to the stems, cover and leave for two days. Then place the stems and the syrup in a pan and bring to a boil again. Preheat an oven to 200°F (100°C) and place the stems (after sprinkling with confectioners' sugar) on a tray until they have completely dried out. Store in an airtight jar.*

WARNING: Avoid during pregnancy as large doses of angelica may disrupt blood pressure. This herb should also be avoided by people who suffer from high blood pressure. Some people suffer sunlight sensitivity due to a substance called furocoumarin, which may also cause skin irritation.

ROMAN CHAMOMILE

Anthemis nobilis

T HE ANCIENT EGYPTIANS make reference to the use of chamomile in their writings, making it another herb with a long and trusted history.

Chamomile has been taken for centuries to calm the nerves and induce rest. When taken internally, the herb assists in soothing an upset stomach and menstrual cramps and dulling muscular aches and travel sickness, as chamomile has an excellent antispasmodic action.

Chamomile tea can be drunk to help reduce nasal congestion and lower temperatures associated with colds and flu. A tincture is especially useful for childhood teething problems, as chamomile has natural painkilling properties. It is also safe to use for children. Chamomile is an excellent antiseptic and can help to relieve urinary infections, including cystitis. The best method is to drink copious amounts of chamomile tea, sit in a chamomile bath and place hot compresses on the lower abdomen. Chamomile is also a mild diuretic which helps reduce fluid retention. This may be helpful in premenstrual syndrome as it may alleviate bloating. This herb is a good antidepressant and may relieve anxiety and tension. An aromatherapy application may be beneficial for helping depression.

An external application rapidly soothes sunburn, hemorrhoids, skin wounds, mastitis and skin ulcers. An immune-stimulating action has also been reported.

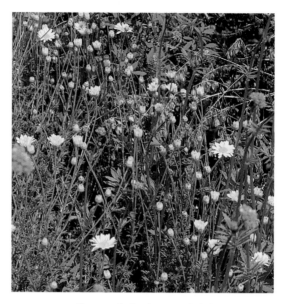

*Chamomile (*Anthemis nobilis*)*

PARTS USED
🌢 *Flowers and essential oil*

DOSAGE
🌢 *As a tincture, take 15–20 drops twice daily.*
🌢 *As a tea, follow the manufacturer's instructions.*
🌢 *As an aromatherapy application, use 6 drops essential oil mixed with 2 teaspoons (10 ml) of almond oil. Massage in the usual way.*
🌢 *For external application, use as a cream or compress.*

POTENTIAL BENEFITS
🌢 *Calms the nerves*
🌢 *Reduces internal inflammation, especially of the stomach, and reduces flatulence*
🌢 *Aids in teething pain*
🌢 *Helps reduce nasal congestion*
🌢 *Soothes irritated skin and skin wounds*
🌢 *Eases menstrual cramps*

COSMETIC USES
🌢 *Chamomile can be used in a cleansing milk for dry and chapped skin and in a shampoo for fair hair. It is also useful as a hand cream. A few drops of chamomile oil can be added for a relaxing bath.*

WARNING: Avoid using the essential oil during early pregnancy as it can stimulate menstruation.

CELERY

Apium graveolens

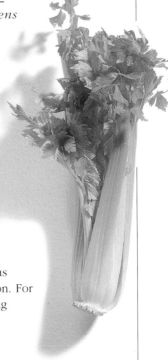

CELERY WAS PRESENT in the tomb of Tutankhamen (c. 1370–1352 B.C.) and has been used as a food and spice for as long as records have been kept.

Celery can reduce blood pressure probably as a result of its diuretic action. Inflammation of the bladder, gout and arthritis all show improvements when treated with celery extracts. An external application helps in cases of fungal infections, and drinking celery juice has been reported to stimulate menstruation. For this reason its use is not advised during pregnancy.

PARTS USED
❦ *Whole plant*

DOSAGE
❦ *Drink a small tumbler or ⅔ cup (150 ml/¼ pint) of fresh juice daily (best diluted 50:50 with water).*
❦ *Add 5 drops of oil extract to a tumbler or ⅔ cup (150 ml/¼ pint) of water daily.*
❦ *For external application, add 6 drops of essential oil to 2 teaspoons (10 ml) almond oil and massage into the area twice a day to eradicate fungal infections.*

POTENTIAL BENEFITS
❦ *Acts as a diuretic*
❦ *Has anti-inflammatory properties*
❦ *Promotes menstruation*
❦ *Reduces arthritis symptoms*

CULINARY USES
❦ *Celery can be washed, and eaten raw.*

WARNING: Avoid concentrated extracts or tinctures during pregnancy.

BURDOCK

Arctium lappa

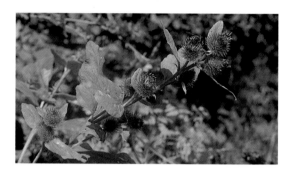

URDOCK HAS SWEET roots and bitter leaves. The roots contain a mucilaginous substance that has a calming and anti-inflammatory action on the stomach.

In herbal medicine burdock has traditionally been used internally for the treatment of psoriasis, eczema, rheumatism and gout. In Chinese medicine, burdock was said to be of benefit in treating pneumonia and throat infections. Burdock also acts as a mild diuretic and detoxifying agent in chronic diseases such as arthritis.

Externally burdock can be very soothing when applied to eczema or other inflammatory skin conditions.

PARTS USED
❦ *Roots, stems and seeds*

DOSAGE
❦ *As a liquid tincture, take 15 drops twice daily.*
❦ *For external application, apply as a cream, compress or poultice as required.*

POTENTIAL BENEFITS
❦ *Acts as a mild diuretic*
❦ *Has a detoxifying action*
❦ *Soothes skin irritations*
❦ *Reduces muscular stiffness associated with rheumatism*
❦ *Controls blood sugar levels*
❦ *Stimulates the immune system*

CULINARY USES
❦ *Burdock root can be cooked like carrots, or the stalks of the young leaves can be scraped and eaten like celery.*

UVA-URSI (BEARBERRY OR UPLAND CRANBERRY)

Arctostaphylos uva-ursi

THE BACTERIUM *E. coli* is very susceptible to the chemicals found in uva-ursi. The antibacterial agent arbutin has given this herb a special place in the treatment of urinary tract infections, especially cystitis. In addition to its antibiotic activity, the herb has a beneficial diuretic action that helps in the elimination of the infective agent. In addition, uva-ursi has high astringent actions that can help relieve minor vaginal infections.

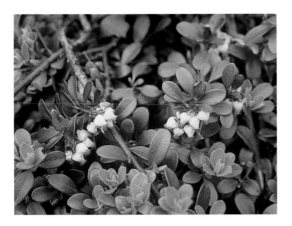

PARTS USED
❦ *Leaves*

DOSAGE
❦ *Take 2 tablets (100 mg) of dried herb daily until symptoms are relieved.*
❦ *As a douche, infuse 1 tablespoon (15 ml) of dried herb, strain and apply.*

POTENTIAL BENEFITS
❦ *Soothes symptoms of bladder and mild kidney infections*
❦ *Acts as a diuretic*
❦ *Relieves minor vaginal infections*
❦ *Reduces symptoms of cystitis*

HORSERADISH

Armoracia rusticana

T HIS VERY AROMATIC herb contains oils that can control microbial infections and even lower fever by increasing perspiration as the volatile oils are eliminated.

It is an excellent remedy for lung infections. During the elimination of the oils from the lung, the antibacterial activity permeates through the entire lung, cleansing as it goes. As a diuretic, horseradish is quite effective, but its stimulating action on digestion is greater. A horseradish poultice has been traditionally used over areas of infection, especially over the chest for the treatment of pleurisy. The drawing properties of horseradish are said to clear the infection.

PARTS USED
❦ *Leaves and roots*

DOSAGE
❦ *For external application, use as a poultice. Add the shredded herb to a mixture of flour and water to make a paste and apply to the area. Cover.*
❦ *As a liquid tincture, take 20 drops twice daily after eating.*
❦ *Mix the shredded herb with honey and hot water for an effective cold remedy.*

POTENTIAL BENEFITS
❦ *Acts as a mild diuretic*
❦ *Cleanses the lungs*
❦ *Acts as an antimicrobial agent*
❦ *Clears infections*
❦ *Stimulates digestion*

CULINARY USES
❦ *Try the fresh leaves in salads or with smoked fish. Roast beef would not be the same without a serving of horseradish sauce.*

ARNICA

Arnica montana

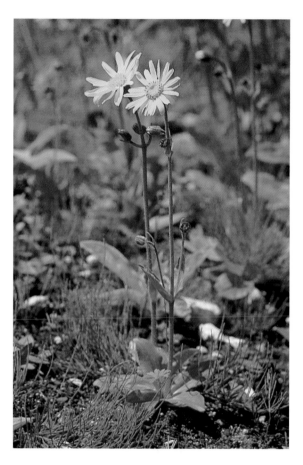

A RNICA ROSE TO fame during the eighteenth century as a cure-all. Although many claims were exaggerated, arnica still holds a special place in herbal medicine today. The plant produces a single, large, yellow flower that lasts throughout the summer. The leaves are picked during the growing season.

Recent studies on arnica have suggested that internal use should be avoided. In the United Kingdom, its external use is widespread. However, short-term internal use, under the supervision of a qualified practitioner, may be helpful for the control of some heart conditions.

When used on the skin, arnica has remarkable properties and can assist the healing process. Bruises, cuts and abrasions all respond very well to arnica cream. Sports injuries, when caught early, improve quickly with an arnica preparation. Arnica liniments are available for the treatment of muscular rheumatism and arthritis.

PARTS USED
🌣 Leaves

DOSAGE
🌣 *Internal use should be undertaken with professional guidance only, but homeopathic preparations containing arnica are considered to be very safe. Try using a 4x or 6x strength tincture remedy at a dose of 5–10 drops taken three times a day about a half hour before eating. Take this remedy with water only.*

🌣 *For external application, follow the manufacturer's instructions.*

POTENTIAL BENEFITS
🌣 *Reduces inflammation in tissues*
🌣 *Stimulates the healing process*
🌣 *Reduces muscular spasm and joint inflammation*
🌣 *Soothes irritated skin*

COSMETIC USES
🌣 *Can be made into creams to stimulate the skin's circulation.*

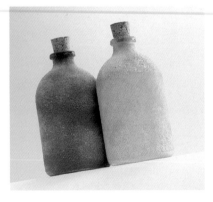

WARNING: Avoid during pregnancy. Do not take internally unless under professional advice as an overdose can prove fatal. External use may cause skin irritation. Never apply to broken skin.

SOUTHERNWOOD

Artemisia abrotanum

T HE PLANT'S USE dates back to ancient
China, where it was used externally for
the treatment of inflamed or burned skin.
The herb is very bitter, and its effectiveness
can be ascribed to the high concentrations of
astringents present in the plant extracts. This
plant has a tonic effect
on the digestive
system. An
improved bile and
digestive juice flow
can be noted after its
use. The muscles of
the uterus can react
strongly to this botanical
substance, and menstruation
can be induced by taking the
extract. For this reason, it must
never be taken during pregnancy.
This herb has also been reported
to help in expelling worms in
children.

PARTS USED
❦ *Leaves*

DOSAGE
❦ *As a liquid tincture, take 20
drops daily.*
❦ *For external application, use
as a compress for irritated skin.*

POTENTIAL BENEFITS
❦ *Stimulates digestion*
❦ *Aids in the flow of bile and,
therefore, the digestion of fat*
❦ *Helps in painful
menstruation*
❦ *Soothes irritated skin*
❦ *Helps expel worms in
children*

WARNING: Avoid during pregnancy.

ASTRAGALUS

Astragalus membranaceus

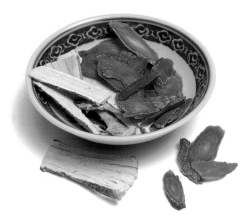

ASTRAGALUS WAS HELD in high esteem by the Chinese, who incorporated it into many of their medicinal formulas. The herb has a sweet taste and has been used in traditional medicine as an immune system, lung, liver and spleen stimulator. It also stimulates the circulatory system and acts as a heart tonic. Beneficial effects of lowering high blood pressure and blood glucose levels have also been reported.

Herbal practitioners may suggest using this herb during treatment with chemotherapy as it stimulates the immune system, but this approach needs cooperation between the herbalist and doctor and should not be taken without supervision.

PART USED
❦ Root

DOSAGE
❦ As a liquid tincture, take 15–20 drops daily.

POTENTIAL BENEFITS
❦ Has a general tonic effect
❦ May help lower blood glucose levels
❦ Stimulates the immune system
❦ Aids the flow of bile and liver function
❦ May help lower blood pressure

OATS

Avena sativa

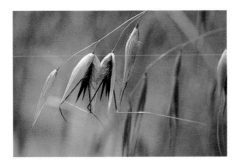

OATS CAN BE considered a food as well as an herb. Oats are a rich source of vitamins (especially vitamin E), carbohydrates, and protein.

The heart, nerves and thymus glands all benefit from a dose of oats. The high silica content makes oats a good food to eat if your cholesterol level is high.

As a remedy for exhaustion, oats act as a nutritive nervine or nerve tonic and may help in cases of depression. For eczema, oats form a good poultice, which helps reduce inflammation and irritation.

PARTS USED
❦ Seeds

DOSAGE
❦ As a liquid tincture, take 25 drops twice daily.
❦ For external application, use as a poultice. Mix oats into a thick, sticky mass with a little hot water and apply to the skin.

POTENTIAL BENEFITS
❦ Acts as a heart and nerve tonic

❦ Lowers cholesterol levels
❦ May help relieve depression
❦ Eases symptoms of eczema

COSMETIC USES
❦ Use oatmeal for facial scrubs to cleanse the skin

CULINARY USES
❦ Cooked oats are made into oatmeal. Oats can form the basis for pancakes.

BORAGE

Borago officinalis

A FAMILIAR HERB to cooks, borage has been associated with mood-enhancing effects. The exact constituents of this plant have not been identified, but its reputation for "lifting the spirits" dates back to 1597, when John Gerard included it in his book *The Herball, or Generall Historie of Plantes*. In this book, borage was said to "drive away sorrow and increase the joy of the mind." During this time, the leaves and flowers were often made into wines and given to men and women to make them "glad and merry." Borage has a very high GLA (gamma linoleic acid) content— higher than evening primrose oil (*Oenothera biennis*)—which helps reduce menstrual cramps. Borage tea is said to be good for lowering high temperatures as it has an excellent diaphoretic action. This makes it an ideal remedy for relieving cold and flu symptoms.

PARTS USED
❦ *Leaves, flowers, oil and seeds*

DOSAGE
❦ *As a liquid tincture, take 15–20 drops twice daily.*
❦ *Borage oil can be taken at a dose of 500 mg daily.*
❦ *As a tea, add about 2 teaspoons (10 ml) of herbs to 2½ cups (600 ml/1 pint) of boiling water and infuse for 5 minutes.*

POTENTIAL BENEFITS
❦ *Has mood-lifting effects*
❦ *Helps in cases of premenstrual tension*
❦ *Helps dermatitis and other skin irritations such as eczema*
❦ *Lowers high temperatures*

CULINARY USES
❦ *Try adding chopped borage to vegetables and pasta dishes, or sprinkle the leaves on salads as a garnish.*

CALENDULA

Calendula officinalis

ALSO KNOWN AS marigold, calendula has a long history in herbal medicine. Initially used to dye fabric, as a food and in cosmetics, calendula contains many oils that have health-promoting properties. Used externally, calendula can reduce inflamed skin and sunburn and promote the healing of wounds. It can also be used to relieve cracked

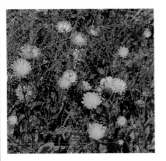

nipples when breast-feeding. The oil can reduce earache.

Its internal use can help stomach ulcers and inflammation. Studies have confirmed the effectiveness of calendula in treating menstrual cramps.

PARTS USED
❦ *Flower petals*

DOSAGE
❦ *As a tea, follow manufacturer's directions.*
❦ *As a liquid tincture, take 15 drops twice daily.*
❦ *For external application, use as a cream, compress or poultice for wounds and inflamed skin as needed.*

POTENTIAL BENEFITS
❦ *Reduces inflammation*
❦ *Eases menstrual cramps*
❦ *Soothes irritated and damaged skin, such as minor burns*
❦ *Relieves earache*

COSMETIC USES
❦ *May be used in a cream to help dry and irritated skin and sore or cracked nipples.*
❦ *The petals can be used in the bath to cleanse and tone the skin.*

CAYENNE

Capsicum frutescens

THERE HAS BEEN much interest in cayenne since it was shown to reduce sensitivity to pain. Cayenne has the ability to overstimulate nerves and deplete their stores of chemicals that relay information to the brain. In effect, the nerves cannot send pain messages. Cayenne has been used medicinally (externally as a cream) to treat chronic pain syndromes such as post-shingles neuralgia and osteoarthritis. Cayenne contains liberal amounts of vitamins, especially the B complex, and it has more vitamin C than an orange. This herb has beneficial effects on the blood's fat content by reducing the levels of low-density lipoprotein (bad cholesterol) and triglycerides.

Cayenne has the ability to stimulate the circulatory system and can be used to treat varicose veins. This herb is also used to treat asthma and pleurisy. It stimulates the release of adrenaline that opens up the airways. It should always be used with caution and always under supervision.

PARTS USED
❧ Fruits

DOSAGE
❧ *Take 1 or 2 tablets (100 mg) of dried herb with a meal.*
❧ *For external application, apply cream daily for no longer than 1 month.*

POTENTIAL BENEFITS
❧ *Relieves pain in cases of chronic neuralgia (external use)*
❧ *Reduces pain of osteoarthritis*
❧ *Stimulates digestion*
❧ *Stimulates circulation*
❧ *Protects the heart from excessive cholesterol*
❧ *May relieve pleurisy*
❧ *Eases varicose vein symptoms*

WARNING: Do not apply cream to broken skin.

PAW PAW

Carica papaya

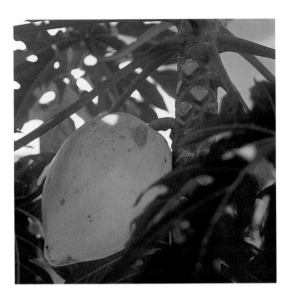

THIS IS NATURE'S very best digestive aid. The enzymes contained in pawpaw break down proteins very efficiently. If you find that you bloat after eating, try some pawpaw after a meal.

As a remedy for intestinal worms (threadworms and roundworms), pawpaw works in almost all cases.

The papain content of pawpaw can help speed wound healing and soften scar tissue.

PARTS USED
❧ *Leaves, fruits, seeds and sap*

DOSAGE
❧ *For a worm remedy, take 2 tablets (50 mg) of dried extract daily.*
❧ *For a digestive aid, take the tablets during every meal or drink fresh juice after each meal.*

POTENTIAL BENEFITS
❧ *Aids digestion*
❧ *Relieves abdominal bloating after eating*
❧ *Helps eliminate worms*

CARAWAY

Carum carvi

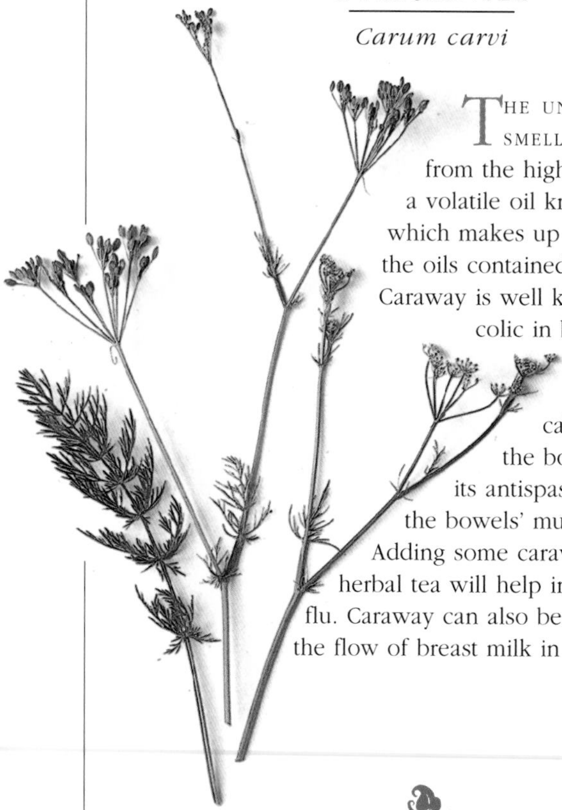

THE UNMISTAKABLE SMELL of caraway comes from the high concentration of a volatile oil known as carvone, which makes up 40–60 percent of the oils contained within the seeds. Caraway is well known for reducing colic in babies and flatulence in adults. Its calming effect on the bowels is based on its antispasmodic activity on the bowels' muscular wall. Adding some caraway seeds to an herbal tea will help in fighting a cold or flu. Caraway can also be used to stimulate the flow of breast milk in nursing mothers.

PARTS USED

- *Seeds, leaves, roots and oil extract*

DOSAGE

- *Add a pinch of seeds to an herbal tea.*
- *Add 2 or 3 drops of infant colic formula to each feeding to combat colic.*

POTENTIAL BENEFITS

- *Eases colic in babies*
- *Reduces flatulence and aids digestion in adults*
- *Helps fight colds, flu and bronchitis*
- *Stimulates the flow of breast milk*

CULINARY USES

- *Try adding caraway seeds to cooking water for vegetables. Add to cheese fondues, bread mixes and goulash. It is good when added to lentil dishes.*

CENTAURY

Centaurium erythraea

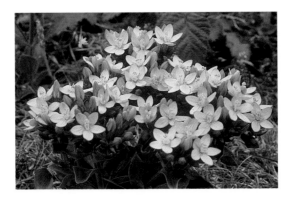

GROWING IN LARGE numbers in very dry and grassy places, centaury is easily spotted by its characteristic spiky appearance.

All parts of this bitter-tasting plant are used in herbal medicine, especially the stems. A liquid extract of centaury still tastes bitter even after it is diluted 3,500 times!

As a medicine, centaury has general tonic properties, but its most important function is the stimulation of stomach activity and the secretion of gastric juices. It can also be used to relieve dyspepsia, stimulate the appetite and aid in poor digestion. If taken in large doses, it can have a laxative effect.

PARTS USED
❧ *Whole plant*

DOSAGE
❧ *As a liquid tincture, take 25 drops before each meal.*

POTENTIAL BENEFITS
❧ *Stimulates appetite*
❧ *Aids poor digestion*
❧ *Helps reduce stomach gas formation*
❧ *Relieves dyspepsia*
❧ *Has laxative effects in large doses*

GOTU KOLA

Centella asiatica

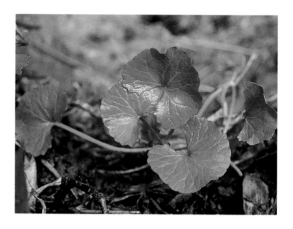

Fɪʀsᴛ ᴜsᴇᴅ ʙʏ Ayurvedic healers in India, this herb has played an important role in controlling the symptoms of stress by inducing a state of relaxation by acting on the nervous system. It acts like a nerve tonic.

Similar to ginkgo (*Ginkgo biloba*), gotu kola stimulates the circulatory system, bringing blood to all parts of the body and stabilizing the cells that make up the walls of the blood vessels. This herb has been shown to improve immune function and stimulate resistance to infection.

Pᴀʀᴛs ᴜsᴇᴅ
🌿 *Whole plant*

Dᴏsᴀɢᴇ
🌿 *Take up to 2 tablets (100 mg) of dried extract daily.*

Pᴏᴛᴇɴᴛɪᴀʟ ʙᴇɴᴇғɪᴛs
🌿 *Improves resistance to disease*
🌿 *Induces a state of relaxation*
🌿 *Relaxes the nervous system*
🌿 *Stimulates circulation to the entire body*

Wᴀʀɴɪɴɢ: Avoid during pregnancy. Do not use if you have an overactive thyroid gland.

BLACK COHOSH

Cimicifuga racemosa

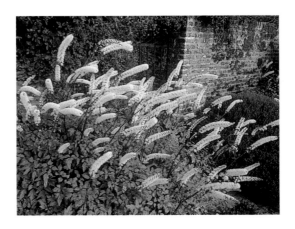

KNOWN AS SQUATROOT by Native Americans who used it for feminine problems, black cohosh can be traced back to the *sheng ma*, a traditional Chinese medical text (c. 25–200 A.D.). It can be used for digestive problems and to soothe arthritic aches and pains. A stimulant effect on the uterus has been noted, so it should not be used during pregnancy. Other uses include treating bronchitis and nausea associated with headaches.

PARTS USED
❦ *Rhizome, for medicinal preparations*

DOSAGE
❦ *Take 1 or 2 tablets (50 mg) of dried herb daily.*
❦ *As a liquid tincture, take 20 drops twice daily.*

POTENTIAL BENEFITS
❦ *Reduces muscular discomfort associated with arthritis*
❦ *Calms menstrual cramps*
❦ *May be helpful in chronic bronchitis*
❦ *Reduces nausea associated with headaches*

WARNING: Because of the stimulant effect on the uterine muscles, avoid during pregnancy.

MYRRH

Commiphora molmol

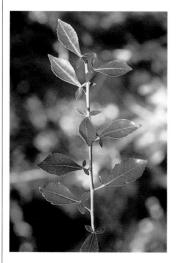

EVER SINCE BIBLICAL times, myrrh has been an essential and standard medicine used in the Middle East for the treatment of wounds, infections and digestive problems. It is especially associated with women's health and purification.

Myrrh has the ability to stimulate healing and reduce inflammation. Its antiseptic properties make it an effective wound cleanser.

Taken internally with echinacea (*Echinacea purpura*), it can speed recovery from infections, especially chest infections, as it has good expectorant and decongestant properties. Myrrh is often taken for relieving colds and bronchitis. When used as a mouthwash, myrrh can strengthen the gums and reduce gum infection and inflammation.

PARTS USED
❦ *Gum resin*

DOSAGE
❦ *As a mouthwash, add 5 drops to a little water.*
❦ *As a liquid tincture, take 10 drops daily.*

POTENTIAL BENEFITS
❦ *Fights gum infections*
❦ *Acts as a wound-cleansing agent*
❦ *Helps fight chest infections*
❦ *Reduces bruising*

WARNING: Do not take myrrh in high doses during pregnancy.

CILANTRO

Coriandrum sativum

CILANTRO HAS BEEN used as a culinary and medicinal herb throughout the centuries. Taken internally, this herb is used to aid digestion and to stimulate the appetite. It also reduces flatulence and helps relieve colic. Cilantro can be especially helpful in reducing diarrhea in children.

As an external application, the lightly bruised seeds can be used as a poultice to alleviate painful joints and rheumatic symptoms.

PARTS USED
❦ *Leaves and seeds*

DOSAGE
❦ *As an infusion, add 1 teaspoon (5 ml) of crushed seeds to 1 cup (250 ml/8 fl oz) of boiling water and let stand for 5 minutes.*
❦ *To relieve flatulence, drink the tea before eating.*
❦ *For external application, use the seeds as a poultice for painful joints.*

POTENTIAL BENEFITS
❦ *Aids digestion*
❦ *Stimulates the appetite*
❦ *Relieves flatulence*
❦ *Reduces diarrhea*
❦ *Helps painful joints*

CULINARY USES
❦ *Use fresh leaves on poultry dishes and add to green salads. Alternatively, use as an ingredient in salad dressings. To make chile-and-cilantro vinaigrette, whisk together three green chilies, deseeded and chopped, ½ teaspoon (2.5 ml) of ground cumin, 3 tablespoons (40 ml) of cider vinegar and salt. Slowly pour in ½ cup (125 ml/4 fl oz) of peanut oil, whisking until well emulsified. Stir in chopped cilantro leaves before serving.*

HAWTHORN

Crataegus oxyacantha

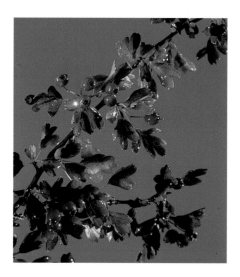

THE BERRIES FROM this plant have been used for digestive problems by herbalists for many years. Its activity on the heart has been likened to that of a heart tonic. The heart benefits in a number of ways. First, the heartbeat is strengthened, which aids a failing heart. Second, the blood vessels are dilated, which reduces the blood pressure and the resultant strain on the heart. Hawthorn has a diuretic action on the body, ridding it of the excess fluid commonly retained by those with heart problems. The hawthorn berries are rich in vitamin C and bioflavonoids—essential factors for blood vessel strength and health.

PARTS USED
❧ *Fruits*

DOSAGE
❧ *As a liquid tincture, take 20 drops twice daily.*

POTENTIAL BENEFITS
❧ *May be used as a heart tonic*
❧ *Increases efficiency of the heartbeat*
❧ *Reduces blood pressure*
❧ *Acts as a diuretic*

TURMERIC
Curcuma longa

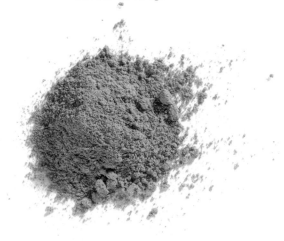

THIS IS A classically pungent herb that forms the basis of most curry powders. Its ability to treat stomach problems effectively has been known for centuries in Asia but only recently in the United States and Europe. Turmeric has the ability to stimulate the flow of bile and, therefore, promote the digestion of fats effectively.

Turmeric has beneficial effects on the circulation, increasing peripheral distribution of blood and helping reduce the incidence of clots. It may also help in menstrual problems, especially in congestive types of premenstrual syndrome, by helping the flow of blood.

PART USED
❦ *Rhizome*

DOSAGE
❦ *Take 2 tablets (50 mg) of dried herb daily after eating.*

POTENTIAL BENEFITS
❦ *Increases circulation*

❦ *Reduces blood clots*
❦ *May help in menstrual problems*
❦ *Stimulates bile flow*
❦ *Aids in fat digestion*

CULINARY USES
❦ *Forms the basis of most curries and curry powders.*

ARTICHOKE

Cynara scolymus

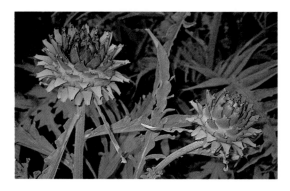

MUCH PRIZED BY the Romans and Greeks, the artichoke has been used for medicinal purposes for centuries. The discovery of a substance called cynarin, which is contained in the leaves, supported the age-old tradition of taking artichoke for problems relating to digestion. Cynarin appears to improve the flow of bile and thus improve the liver function. A secondary effect is a reduction in cholesterol levels due to the increased flow of bile.

PARTS USED
❧ *Flower heads, leaves and roots*

DOSAGE
❧ *As a liquid tincture, take 20 drops twice daily.*

POTENTIAL BENEFITS
❧ *Stimulates the flow of digestive juices*
❧ *Increases bile flow*
❧ *Promotes liver function*
❧ *Reduces cholesterol levels*

CULINARY USES
❧ *There is nothing nicer than artichoke vinaigrette. Place an unopened flower head in a pan of boiling water. Reduce the heat and cook for about 15 minutes or until the leaves can be pulled off easily. Drain well, place on a small serving plate and drizzle a vinaigrette dressing over the leaves. Serve immediately.*

ECHINACEA

Echinacea purpura

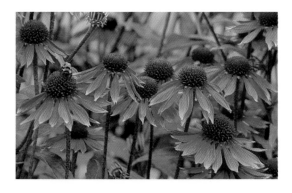

THE HEDGEHOG-LIKE appearance of the central cone of echinacea, or purple coneflower, gave this herb its name, from the Greek *echinos* meaning "hedgehog." Echinacea is probably one of the most commonly used herbal extracts today. In Germany, the liquid extract is referred to as "resistance drops," owing to echinacea's immune-stimulating effect.

Externally, echinacea can be used to heal minor cuts and scrapes. For all problems relating to bacterial, fungal or viral infection, echinacea should be the first herb of choice.

PARTS USED
❦ *Roots and rhizomes*

DOSAGE
❦ *In acute illness, take up to 40 drops (20 for children) of liquid tincture every four hours.*
❦ *For prevention of colds and flu, take 10–15 drops daily.*
❦ *In tablet form, take 1 or 2 tablets (50–100 mg) of dried extract daily.*

❦ *For external application, use as a cream for cuts and scrapes.*

POTENTIAL BENEFITS
❦ *Stimulates the immune system*
❦ *Prevents the progression of infections*
❦ *Relieves symptoms of colds and flu, especially when nasal congestion is a problem*
❦ *Has a virus killing action*

GINSENG (SIBERIAN)

Eleutherococcus senticosus

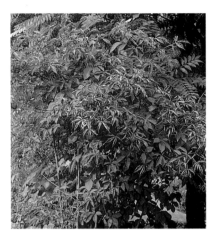

THE ACTIVE AGENTS of Siberian ginseng are similar to the *Panax* ginseng form but are considered to be less potent. Siberian ginseng can be taken for longer periods than the *Panax* ginseng form and is thought to be better suited to the treatment of stress when an extended treatment program is needed. It may also be used to improve physical and mental stamina. There are claims that it may reduce cholesterol and blood sugar levels.

PARTS USED
- Roots

DOSAGE
- *Take 2 teaspoons (10 ml) of ginseng elixir daily.*

POTENTIAL BENEFITS
- *Improves resistance to stress*
- *Increases mental agility*
- *May reduce cholesterol and blood sugar levels*

WARNING: Generally, ginseng should not be used continuously for longer than 1 month.

HORSETAIL

Equisetum arvense

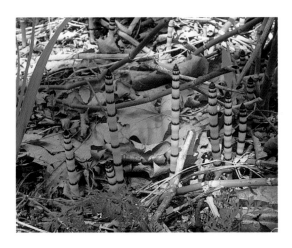

CONTAINED WITHIN THIS herb is an interesting cocktail of nutrients and phytochemicals. Horsetail is rich in silica and other minerals that facilitate the absorption of calcium from the diet. Nails and hair greatly benefit from this herb, as do the bones and other connective tissues that depend on calcium and trace minerals for their health. Its high silica content may help reduce cholesterol levels.

Horsetail may help regulate the skin's oil production, which in turn may help reduce outbreaks of acne and other congestive skin blemishes.

PARTS USED
☙ *Stems*

DOSAGE
☙ *As a liquid tincture, take 15–20 drops twice daily.*

POTENTIAL BENEFITS
☙ *Adds strength to nails and hair*
☙ *Supports healthy bone and tissue development*
☙ *Helps reduce acne in those with oily skin*
☙ *May help reduce cholesterol levels*

CALIFORNIAN POPPY

Eschscholzia californica

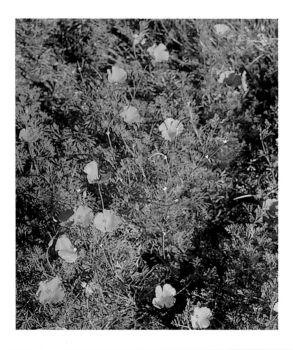

THE WATERY SAP of this plant has a mild painkilling action. The Native Americans often used this to reduce the pain of toothache. The action of this plant appears to be in the central nervous system and is thought to be narcotic in nature. It has also been used as a sedative and may help insomnia.

PARTS USED
❧ *Whole plant*

DOSAGE
❧ *As a liquid tincture, take 5–10 drops as needed.*

POTENTIAL BENEFITS
❧ *Has a painkilling action if applied topically in cases of toothache*
❧ *Reduces anxiety and tension when used internally*
❧ *May help insomnia*

EUCALYPTUS

Eucalyptus globulus

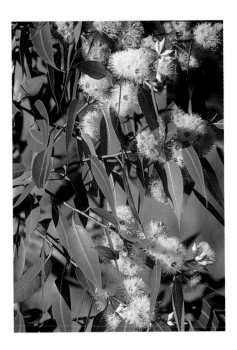

T HERE ARE MORE than 40 different types of eucalyptus
trees, all of which are rich in the volatile oils that are
responsible for the aroma.

Traditional aboriginal uses are well-kept secrets, but it was
known to help treat dysentery. The extracts from eucalyptus
have a great decongestant action due to the high content of
aromatic oils. Eucalyptus, also called the blue gum tree, can
help in expectoration because it acts as a respiratory stimulant.

Used externally, eucalyptus can help heal sports injuries.
Eucalyptus has an antiseptic action that helps reduce muscle
spasm. Muscular aches and pains benefit greatly from an
application of a eucalyptus-based cream or lotion.

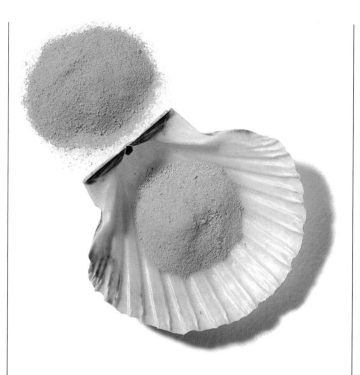

PARTS USED
❧ *Leaves and essential oils*

DOSAGE
❧ *As a vapor inhalant, use about 4 drops in a vaporizer and inhale for about 5 minutes.*
❧ *For external application, use as a cream or lotion, as required.*

POTENTIAL BENEFITS
❧ *Acts as a decongestant for upper respiratory infections*
❧ *Clears sinus congestion*
❧ *Stimulates the removal of lung congestion*
❧ *Has an antimicrobial activity*
❧ *Can be used as an effective muscle ointment*

COSMETIC USES
❧ *Can be used in a lotion or skin tonic to stimulate the skin's circulation.*
❧ *Add a couple of drops of essential oil to a bath to soothe aching muscles.*

WARNING: Do not use on open wounds. Avoid excessive exposure to vapors, as eucalyptus can cause headaches and may aggravate asthma symptoms.

EYEBRIGHT

Euphrasis officinalis

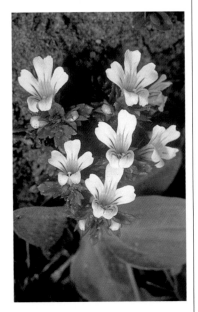

THROUGH THE DOCTRINE of Signatures (if the appearance of the plant or flower looks like an anatomical part, then the herb will help diseases of that area), eyebright became a cure-all for eye problems. The flowers have purple and yellow stripes and spots that resemble the human iris.

The astringent properties of eyebright do make it a useful herb for the treatment of sore and inflamed eyes (conjunctivitis) and other irritant eye problems such as weeping eczema which can occur around the eyes as well as ultra-sensitivity to light.

PARTS USED
❦ *Whole plant*

DOSAGE
❦ *For an eye bath, use a commercially made preparation to minimize the risk of infection.*

❦ *As a liquid tincture, take 1 or 2 drops twice daily.*

POTENTIAL BENEFITS
❦ *Calms irritated eyes and helps reduce conjunctivitis*
❦ *Promotes good eye health when taken internally*

WARNING: Avoid high doses of eyebright during pregnancy.

FENNEL

Foeniculum vulgare

FRESH FENNEL DELIVERS a special aroma due to the two oils, anethole and fenchone, which vary from species to species. Taken internally, fennel aids the digestive process and soothes cases of colic and abdominal discomfort. It can be taken in the form of a tea or as "fennel water," which is very easy to make. It is thought that if this is drunk during breast-feeding it will help reduce colic and act as a general digestive aid. Fennel also has a mild diuretic action and a cleansing action on the kidneys. It can promote the flow of breast milk in nursing mothers.

PARTS USED
🍂 *Leaves, stems, roots and seeds*

DOSAGE
🍂 *As a liquid tincture, take 20 drops just after eating.*
🍂 *As fennel water, put about 2 pinches of fennel seeds in 1 cup (250 ml/8 fl oz) of water and bring to a boil. As the water starts to change color, keep boiling for 1 minute. Strain and cool before drinking. Keep in the refrigerator.*
🍂 *As a tea, add 2 teaspoons of seeds to 1 cup (250 ml/8 fl oz) of boiling water and let stand for 5 minutes.*

POTENTIAL BENEFITS
🍂 *Acts as a digestive aid*
🍂 *Reduces abdominal cramping and colic*
🍂 *Reduces flatulence*
🍂 *Acts as a remedy for infantile colic*
🍂 *Acts as a mild diuretic and kidney cleanser*
🍂 *Promotes flow of breast milk in nursing mothers*

COSMETIC USES
🍂 *The seeds can be used in a lotion to help oily skin.*

CULINARY USES
🍂 *Try fennel seeds in fish dishes or use during the cooking of vegetables. Fresh fennel bulb can be cooked whole and eaten as a vegetable. It has a wonderful aniseed flavor and is a good accompaniment with poultry and lamb.*

WARNING: Avoid during pregnancy.

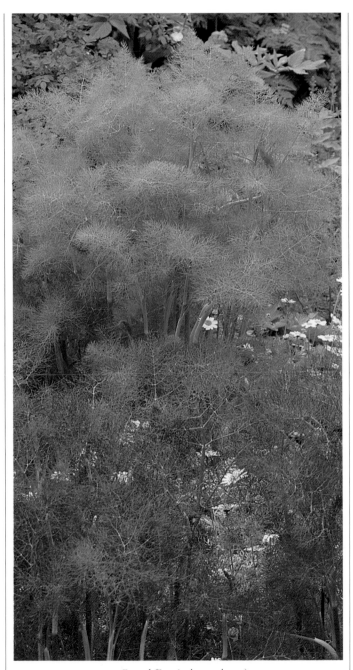

Fennel (Foeniculum vulgare*)*

AMERICAN CRANESBILL

Geranium maculatum

THIS HERB IS known to be a common medicine used by Native Americans for the treatment of diarrhea and stomach complaints. Analysis of the plant extracts shows a high concentration of astringents. A traditional use of this plant is the control of excessive bleeding associated with menstruation. A topical application of the plant is applied to infected wounds, thrush and hemorrhoids.

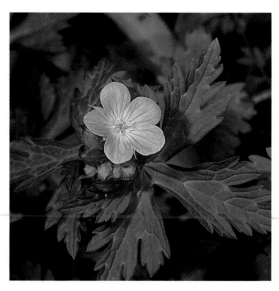

PARTS USED
- *Whole plant*

DOSAGE
- *As a liquid tincture, take 20–25 drops twice daily.*
- *For external application, use as a compress for wounds, thrush and hemorrhoids.*

POTENTIAL BENEFITS
- *Has an antiseptic action*
- *Reduces blood flow in menstruation*
- *Soothes hemorrhoid irritation*
- *Reduces diarrhea*

GINKGO

Ginkgo biloba

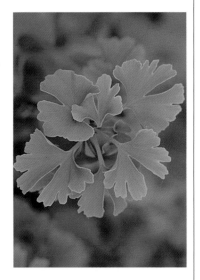

FOSSIL RECORDS SHOW that the ginkgo tree has remained unchanged for millions of years. The trees were present even before mammals walked the earth.

Extracts of the leaves yield a fascinating substance that has profound effects on the allergic response. These chemicals, ginkgolides, act to inhibit platelet-activating factor, a key substance in the allergic response. Other chemicals, ginkgo flavonoids, have a stimulating effect on the blood circulation of the brain and periphery.

Ginkgo has been effectively used for the treatment of asthma, tinnitus, allergic inflammatory conditions and varicose veins. It has also been used to treat reduced brain circulation and Raynaud's disease as this herb improves peripheral circulation. In this disease, peripheral circulation is badly affected, and the hands often turn blue.

PARTS USED
❦ *Leaves and seeds*

DOSAGE
❦ *As a liquid tincture, take 20 drops twice daily.*

POTENTIAL BENEFITS
❦ *Improves blood circulation to the brain*
❦ *Reduces symptoms of tinnitus*
❦ *Reduces allergic conditions*
❦ *Helps in Raynaud's disease*
❦ *May reduce asthma symptoms*

LICORICE

Glycyrrhiza glabra

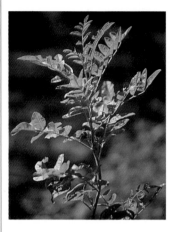

THE MAIN CONSTITUENT of licorice is a substance called glycyrrhizin, which is 50 times sweeter than sugar.

Glycyrrhizin reduces inflammation and has been used in treating menstrual irregularities. Taken 14 days prior to menstruation, licorice can suppress the breakdown of progesterone and improve depression, sugar cravings, water retention and breast tenderness.

Taken internally, licorice can help Addison's disease, as glycyrrhizin has a similar effect to an adrenal hormone called aldosterone. Licorice has a detoxifying action on the liver.

An estrogen-like action has been noted, making it a good remedy for the relief of menopausal symptoms. Taken for stomach problems, licorice has a great healing power on the lining of the stomach.

PARTS USED
- Roots

DOSAGE
- *Chew 2 or 3 tablets (100 mg) with each meal.*

POTENTIAL BENEFITS
- *Speeds the healing of stomach ulcers*
- *Helps in menstrual irregularities*
- *Detoxifies the liver*
- *Helps in Addison's disease*
- *Relieves the symptoms of the menopause*

WARNING: Because of the sodium content of licorice, avoid during pregnancy. Do not use if you have high blood pressure or kidney disease or if you are taking the heart drug Digoxin.

HOPS

Humulus lupulus

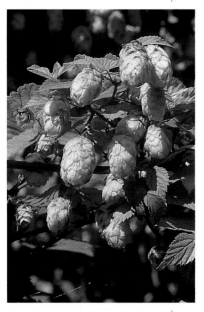

Hops are one of nature's best relaxants. The herb exerts a calming effect on the whole body, relieving nervous tension, irritability and insomnia.

For the treatment of irritable bowel syndrome and a nervous stomach, hops can prove to be a very effective remedy. A good combination is equal parts of valerian (*Valeriana officinalis*) and hops taken about a half hour before bed to induce a natural and restful sleep.

A poultice made from hops can be helpful for cases of eczema and skin ulcerations.

PARTS USED
❦ *Leaves and shoots*

DOSAGE
❦ *As a soothing agent for irritable bowels, take 2 tablets (50 mg) daily.*
❦ *As a sedative, try the mixture described above at bedtime.*
❦ *For external application, use as a poultice for eczema and skin ulcers.*

POTENTIAL BENEFITS
❦ *Acts as a sedative to promote restful sleep*
❦ *Acts as a calming agent for a nervous stomach*
❦ *Relieves irritable bowel syndrome*
❦ *Acts as an anti-stress herb*
❦ *Relieves eczema and skin ulcerations*

CULINARY USES
❦ *The young side shoots can be cooked and eaten.*

WARNING: Avoid if you suffer from depression.

GOLDENSEAL

Hydrastis canadensis

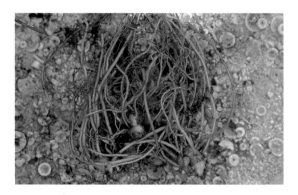

G OLDENSEAL CAN ACT as a double-edged sword. When given for infections of the bowels, it tends to destroy the beneficial bacteria as well as the disease-causing ones. It is recommended, therefore, that its use should be restricted to one month followed by a course of probiotics (capsules containing cultures of good bacteria for the bowel).

Goldenseal can also be used as a laxative. Externally, it can be used for treating irritated skin and conjunctivitis.

PARTS USED
❦ *Rhizomes*

DOSAGE
❦ *As a liquid tincture, take 20 drops daily.*
❦ *For an eyebath, use a commercially made preparation to minimize the risk of infection.*

❦ *For external application, use as a lotion, compress or cream use as required*

POTENTIAL BENEFITS
❦ *Reduces constipation*
❦ *Has an antibacterial action in bowel and gut infections*
❦ *Helps relieve irritated skin*
❦ *Acts as a laxative*

WARNING: Do not use for longer than 1 month. Avoid during pregnancy as goldenseal stimulates the uterine muscles.

ST. JOHN'S WORT

Hypericum perfortum

THERE HAS BEEN much interest in this herb since a study found it to be as effective as regular antidepressants but with none of the accompanying side effects. This action was found to be due to the high concentration of hypericin. This herb produces a lovely red pigment when the leaves are crushed between the fingers, and it is the pigment that contains the active agents. St. John's wort has an effective sedative action and can calm nerves and help relieve insomnia.

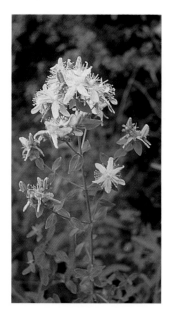

Another interesting aspect to this herb is its ability to stop the multiplication of certain viruses (retroviruses), meaning it may be used to treat AIDS. Used externally as a lotion, St. John's wort has a powerful healing and anti-inflammatory action and can be used to treat varicose veins, bruises and sunburn.

PARTS USED
❧ *Whole plant*

DOSAGE
❧ *As a liquid tincture, take 20 drops twice daily.*
❧ *For external application, use as a lotion as required.*

POTENTIAL BENEFITS
❧ *Acts as a remedy for insomnia*
❧ *Calms nerves*
❧ *Promotes wound-healing*
❧ *Has a potential benefit against AIDS*
❧ *Relieves sunburn*

HYSSOP

Hyssopus officinalis

Hyssop is mentioned in the New Testament of the Bible as an herb that has purification properties. These are largely due to the high content of camphoraceous oils contained within the herb. Its effectiveness in treating lung infections such as bronchitis can be attributed to this substance. It can also be used to relieve coughs, colds and nasal congestion as well as a gargle for sore throats.

Hyssop has the ability to stabilize low blood pressure and prevent the dizzy spells experienced by people with low blood pressure as they rise from a sitting or lying position.

An external application can be used for the treatment of minor cuts and bruises.

PARTS USED
* Whole plant

DOSAGE
* In tablet form, take 2 tablets (50 mg) of dried herb twice daily.
* As a liquid tincture, take 15–20 drops twice daily.
* For external application, use as a compress for minor cuts and bruises.

POTENTIAL BENEFITS
* Stabilizes low blood pressure
* Acts against lung infections
* Helps relieve coughs
* Helps as a topical application for minor cuts and bruises

CULINARY USES
* Try adding a few leaves to meat dishes including beef casseroles. It is also ideal for adding to many legume dishes.

WARNING: The essential oil must be avoided during pregnancy and by people who suffer from epilepsy.

JASMINE

Jasmine officinale

INITIALLY GROWN FOR the perfume industry, jasmine has many possible health-promoting effects. Jasmine has been successfully used for the treatment of sunstroke, fever, irritant dermatitis and infectious illness including coughs. Emotional upsets, post natal depression, premenstrual tension and headaches all respond well to a dose of jasmine as it exhibits powerful antidepressent properties. Jasmine is also very useful for relieving menstrual cramps, as it has the ability to reduce muscular spasms of the uterus. It is regarded as an aphrodisiac when applied to the body in its oil form.

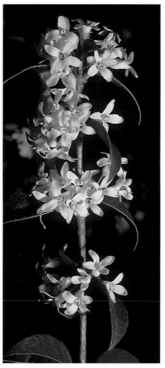

PARTS USED
❦ *Roots, flowers and oil*

DOSAGE
❦ *As a tea, drink 1 cup of jasmine tea daily.*
❦ *For external application, use 6 drops of essential oil mixed with 2 teaspoons (10 ml) of almond oil.*

POTENTIAL BENEFITS
❦ *Improves emotional state*
❦ *May help reduce dermatitis symptoms*
❦ *May act as an aphrodisiac*

COSMETIC USES
❦ *Add 6–8 drops of essential oil for a stimulating bath.*

WARNING: Avoid during early pregnancy.

JUNIPER

Juniperus communis

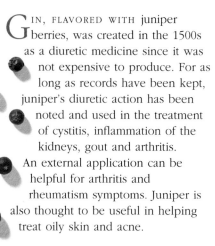

Gin, flavored with juniper berries, was created in the 1500s as a diuretic medicine since it was not expensive to produce. For as long as records have been kept, juniper's diuretic action has been noted and used in the treatment of cystitis, inflammation of the kidneys, gout and arthritis. An external application can be helpful for arthritis and rheumatism symptoms. Juniper is also thought to be useful in helping treat oily skin and acne.

PARTS USED
* *Fruits*

DOSAGE
* *As a liquid tincture, take 20 drops twice daily.*
* *For external application, use 6 drops of juniper berry essential oil in 2 teaspoons (10 ml) of almond oil and massage into arthritic joints.*

POTENTIAL BENEFITS
* *Acts as a powerful diuretic*
* *Reduces symptoms of gout*
* *Aids in cystitis*
* *Soothes joint pains associated with arthritis*

COSMETIC USES
* *May be used in a lotion for oily skin and acne.*

CULINARY USES
* *Add some berries to pâtés, relish or sauerkraut.*

WARNING: Avoid during pregnancy because of the stimulant effect on the muscles of the uterus.

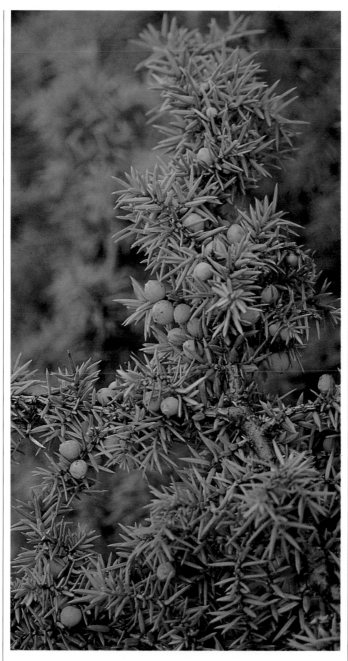

Juniper berries (Juniperus communis)

LAVENDER

Lavandula officinalis

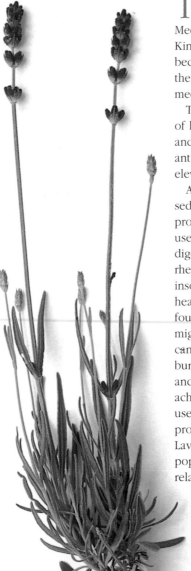

THE ROMANS BROUGHT lavender from the Mediterranean to the United Kingdom. Since then, it has become an essential part of the early monastic and medicinal herb garden.

The aromatic sweet smell of lavender is unmistakable, and it is said to have antidepressant and mood-elevating effects.

As it exhibits powerful sedative and calming properties, lavender has been used for the treatment of digestive problems, anxiety, rheumatism, irritability, insomnia and tension headaches. It has also been found effective for use in migraine headaches. Lavender can be used to treat minor burns, especially sunburn, and rheumatic muscular aches and pains. It is also useful in treating skin problems such as acne. Lavender is one of the most popular essential oils for relaxation.

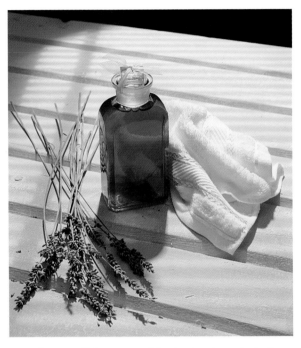

Melt away all the stresses of the day in a lavender bath.

PARTS USED

❦ *Flowers, stems and essential oil*

DOSAGE

❦ *For external application, use 6 drops of essential oil mixed with 2 teaspoons (10 ml) of almond oil to treat the affected area.*
❦ *For a relaxing tea, infuse a commercially prepared tea and drink twice daily.*

POTENTIAL BENEFITS

❦ *Has natural antidepressant effects*
❦ *Acts as a mood elevator*
❦ *Reduces anxiety*
❦ *Helps digestion*
❦ *Soothes rheumatic muscle and joint pains*
❦ *May help relieve migraine headaches*

COSMETIC USES

❦ *Lavender may be used in a lotion for sunburn or in a cream for dry skin.*
❦ *Add 6–8 drops of lavender essential oil for a relaxing bath.*

CULINARY USES

❦ *Try flavoring preserves with lavender or incorporating it into cake and cookie mixes.*

LINSEED OR COMMON FLAX

Linum usitatissimum

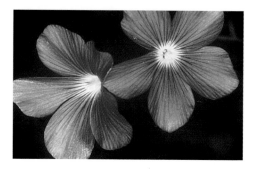

THIS IS GROWN as a farm crop. Contained within this plant are a number of important substances. The oil in the seeds, combined with the plant mucilage, makes an effective laxative. Flax oil on its own has great potential to help reduce the irritation of eczema as it contains high concentrations of essential fatty acids that are needed by the skin. Externally, the crushed seeds can be used in a poultice for treating boils and pleurisy.

PARTS USED
- *Seeds*

DOSAGE
- *As a laxative, chew and swallow 1 or 2 teaspoons (5–10 ml) of seeds at bedtime with a glass of water.*
- *In cases of skin irritation, take 1 or 2 g of flaxseed oil daily after meals.*
- *For external application, use as a poultice made from the crushed seeds for boils and symptoms of pleurisy. Apply to the painful area.*

POTENTIAL BENEFITS
- *Has laxative properties, helpful in chronic constipation*
- *Has an anti-inflammatory action, especially in skin problems such as eczema*
- *Relieves boils*

CULINARY USES
- *Flax flour can be obtained from health food stores and makes great bread.*

DEVIL'S CLAW

Martynia annua

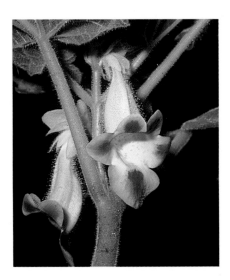

A N EXTRACT OF this herb is used by South African farmers, who note that the locals gain great relief from the symptoms of arthritis and rheumatism after drinking a decoction made from the roots of the plant.

The analgesic effect of this herb is accompanied by its anti-inflammatory action, making it the herb of choice for inflammatory joint problems such as arthritis. The herb has also been noted for its digestive stimulant action.

PARTS USED
- *Tubers*

DOSAGE
- *As a liquid tincture, take 20 drops twice daily.*

POTENTIAL BENEFITS
- *Has a natural painkilling anti-inflammatory action*
- *Soothes symptoms of arthritis and joint swelling*
- *Acts as a mild digestive stimulant*

WARNING: Avoid during pregnancy.

ALFALFA
Medicago sativa

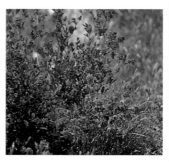

ALFALFA IS AN incredible plant. It can grow in very harsh conditions and transform barren land into a lush pasture. The nutrient content of alfalfa is impressive, comprising vitamins C, D, E, K and the B complex, as well as beta carotene and the minerals potassium, magnesium and calcium. There can be a tendency to consume too much of this herb, but care needs to be taken because it can trigger a flare-up of systemic lupus erythematosus as well as making some people sensitive to sunlight.

Alfalfa is a good laxative and mild diuretic and is used for urinary tract infections. It is given as a tonic for those recovering from any debilitating illness that leaves the patient weak. It has the ability to stimulate the appetite.

PARTS USED
❦ *Whole plant*

DOSAGE
❦ *In tablet form, take up to 5 tablets of dried, compressed alfalfa plant daily.*
❦ *As a liquid tincture, take 15–20 drops twice daily.*

POTENTIAL BENEFITS
❦ *Acts as a diuretic*
❦ *Has a laxative effect*
❦ *Helps recovery from any debilitating illness*
❦ *Helps relieve the symptoms of cystitis*
❦ *Stimulates the appetite*

CULINARY USES
❦ *Seeds can be sprouted and used in salads. Leaves may be eaten raw or cooked.*

WARNING: Do not take if you are suffering from an autoimmune condition such as systemic lupus erythematosus.

LEMON BALM

Melissa officinalis

Tʜɪs ʟᴇᴍᴏɴ-sᴄᴇɴᴛᴇᴅ herb has powerful antiviral and antibacterial effects, which can be helpful in the treatment of recurrent cold sores. An application of a lemon balm-based cream just as the cold sore is forming can prevent it from erupting.

Taken internally, the herb helps with nervous problems and excitability, especially in children. Those who suffer from panic attacks and heart palpitations may find the extract helpful, as the herb has a sedative action and relaxes the nervous system. For the treatment of depression, try an external application of lemon balm in an aromatherapy massage. Some people may prefer an all-over body massage, while others may prefer to have the upper back and shoulders massaged as an anti-stress technique.

Pᴀʀᴛs ᴜsᴇᴅ
❧ *Whole plant*

Dᴏsᴀɢᴇ
❧ *For external application, use as a cream. Apply enough to cover the area three times a day.*
❧ *For aromatherapy application, use 6 drops of oil mixed with 2 teaspoons (10 ml) of almond oil. Massage in the usual way.*
❧ *As a liquid tincture, take 15 drops twice daily.*

Pᴏᴛᴇɴᴛɪᴀʟ ʙᴇɴᴇғɪᴛs
❧ *Has antiviral and antibacterial action*
❧ *Calms the nervous system*
❧ *Helps panic attacks*
❧ *Can help relieve depression*

Cᴏsᴍᴇᴛɪᴄ ᴜsᴇs
❧ *Used in cleansing lotions and as an infusion for relaxing baths.*

Cᴜʟɪɴᴀʀʏ ᴜsᴇs
❧ *Add the leaves to soups, salads and fish dishes. Lemon balm cordial can be purchased. It is similar to an elixir but diluted with water before it is taken. It also forms a vital ingredient in the liqueur Benedictine.*

PEPPERMINT

Mentha piperita

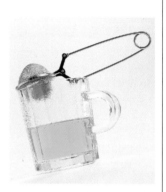

THIS STRONGLY AROMATIC herb has a long history as a decongestant and antiseptic agent and is valuable in the treatment of colds and nasal congestion. The oils contained in the plant have a powerful antispasmodic action on the smooth muscle of the stomach, making it the herb of choice for adult colic, dyspepsia and irritable bowel syndrome.

As a remedy for nausea and morning sickness, the normal internal dose of peppermint is very safe for a pregnant woman. Peppermint is also good for relieving menstrual pain as it has a relaxing effect.

The external application of the oil can help muscular discomfort and neuralgia.

PARTS USED
❧ *Whole plant*

DOSAGE
❧ *2 or 3 commercially prepared capsules (2 ml of oil per capsule) taken between meals to relieve bowel spasms.*
❧ *As a tea, take 1 cup (250 ml/8 fl oz) twice daily.*
❧ *As an aromatherapy massage, use 6 drops of essential oil mixed with 2 teaspoons (10 ml) of almond oil. Massage in the usual way.*

POTENTIAL BENEFITS
❧ *Has an antispasmodic agent for bowels*
❧ *Reduces nausea and sickness associated with early pregnancy*
❧ *Reduces stiffness when used as a muscle rub*
❧ *Has a decongestant action*

CULINARY USES
❧ *Add the leaves to iced tea for a very refreshing drink.*

BASIL

Ocimum basilicum

BASIL IS SOMETIMES referred to as St. Joseph's wort, not to be confused with St. John's wort. Its use dates back to biblical times, when it was seen after the resurrection growing around Christ's tomb. The word "basil" is thought to come from the Greek for "king."

Rich in volatile oils, basil contains over 20 chemical substances, including methyl cinnamate (cinnamon), citral (lemon), thymol (thyme) and camphor. There have been many variants of basil cultivated, each with a different aroma and flavor, making identification of different varieties difficult.

Basil has been taken internally for chills, colds and flu, in which it has a stimulant action. For digestion, basil is of great help in cases of stomach inflammation and helps relieve the abdominal cramps associated with menstruation.

PARTS USED
❧ *Whole plant*

DOSAGE
❧ *As a liquid tincture, take 15 drops twice daily.*

POTENTIAL BENEFITS
❧ *Acts as a stimulant and aids resistance to infection*
❧ *Soothes an inflamed stomach and aids digestion*
❧ *Has an antispasmodic action*

CULINARY USES
❧ *Basil has many uses in cooking. The leaves make a good addition to any salad, adding a special flavor. Basil forms the basis of pesto, a traditional pasta sauce, as well as many stuffings for meat.*

EVENING PRIMROSE

Oenothera biennis

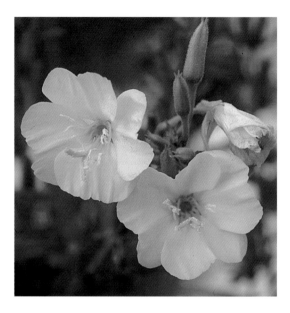

THIS HERB HAS risen to fame as a remedy for premenstrual and menopause symptoms, but there is a lot more to evening primrose than this. It is a very rich source of gamma linoleic acid (GLA), which is an essential fatty acid. GLA is vital for the health of cell membranes and balances the output of hormones. Taking evening primrose oil can block the action of these substances and reduce the discomfort. A dose of this oil can rebalance the hormonal system itself.

The effect on prostaglandins may explain how evening primrose oil can reduce blood pressure and the level of free cholesterol circulating in the blood.

As a remedy for skin problems, evening primrose is safe to use topically on a baby's cradle cap and, should eczema develop, evening primrose can be taken internally.

It is interesting to note that schizophrenia has responded well to evening primrose supplements, although the mechanism behind this is unknown.

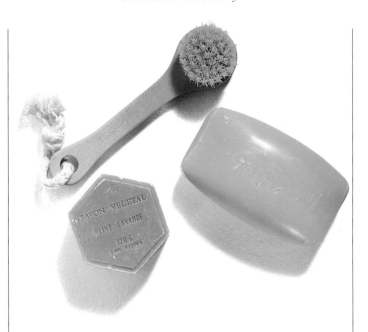

Soap containing evening primrose oil is good for moisturizing the skin.

PARTS USED
❧ Oil

DOSAGE
❧ For menopausal symptoms, take 2 or 3 capsules (500 mg capsules) every evening with water only.
❧ For premenstrual symptoms, take 3 capsules (500 mg capsules) every evening for about 14 days before the onset of menstruation.
❧ For children, use about 250 mg of oil mixed in food daily.
❧ For cradle cap, massage enough to make the area supple.

POTENTIAL BENEFITS
❧ Balances hormones
❧ Acts as an antispasmodic agent for abdominal cramps
❧ Lowers blood pressure
❧ Lowers cholesterol levels
❧ Helps eczema
❧ Helps schizophrenic symptoms

WARNING: Do not use if you suffer from epilepsy or migraines.

OLIVE

Olea europaea

T HE USE OF olive oil in cooking is well known, but for medicinal purposes, extracts are taken from the leaves as well as the fruits themselves. Leaf extracts can be used for the treatment of high blood pressure and nervous tension, while the oil extracted from the fruits aids in cases of constipation.

The heart's health is greatly improved by the use of olive oil (best taken as the cold-pressed extra-virgin type) in cooking and food preparation.

Olive oil has the ability to reduce the bad cholesterol levels without affecting the beneficial cholesterol levels. Because olive oil is monounsaturated, there is little risk of free-radical generation if food is not cooked at very high temperatures.

PARTS USED
❧ *Leaves and fruits*

DOSAGE
❧ *As a laxative, take 2 or 3 tablespoons (30–45 ml) of oil.*
❧ *For general health, use 1 or 2 tablespoons (15–30 ml) mixed with food daily.*

POTENTIAL BENEFITS
❧ *Acts as a heart protector*
❧ *Reduces LDL cholesterol levels*
❧ *Reduces high blood pressure*
❧ *Acts to relax nerves and tension-related problems*
❧ *Helps relieve constipation*

CULINARY USES
❧ *Use the oil for cooking as you would any other oil, but do not cook at very high temperatures. The oil can also be used instead of butter. Chop and use the fruits in pasta sauces and in bread mixes.*

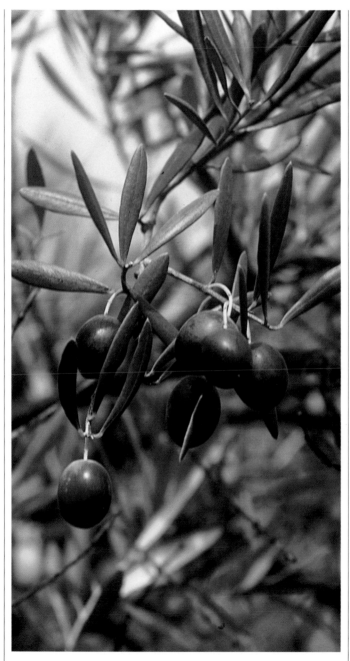

*Olives (*Olea europaea*)*

SWEET MARJORAM

Origanum majorana

THIS IS A popular culinary herb and is used in a variety of dishes. It is used to help digestion and reduce flatulence.

Marjoram is a good antiseptic as it contains a large amount of thymol. It also has a very calming effect on the nerves and is helpful in relieving tension and menstrual cramps. It is helpful when the oil is massaged in an aromatherapy application. Marjoram can be used to soothe sprains and muscular aches and pains. Apply a cold compress to sprains and a hot compress to aches and pains. Marjoram oil can also help with arthritis and rheumatism.

Drinking a marjoram infusion can help fight colds and relieve bronchitis.

Marjoram can give temporary relief from toothache if the leaves are chewed.

PARTS USED
❦ *Leaves and essential oil*

DOSAGE
❦ *As an aromatherapy massage, use 6 drops of essential oil mixed with 2 teaspoons (10 ml) of almond oil. Massage into the skin.*
❦ *As a tea, infuse 2 teaspoons dried leaves in 1 cup (250 ml/ 8 fl oz) of water and let stand for 5 minutes before drinking.*

POTENTIAL BENEFITS
❦ *Aids digestion*
❦ *Relieves tension*
❦ *Helps relieve menstrual cramps*
❦ *Fights colds*
❦ *Relieves arthritis and rheumatism*
❦ *Relieves toothache temporarily*

COSMETIC USES
❦ *Add an infusion of leaves for a relaxing bath.*

CULINARY USES
❦ *Add leaves to casseroles, sauces and egg-and-cheese dishes.*

WARNING: Avoid during pregnancy.

GINSENG

Panax ginseng

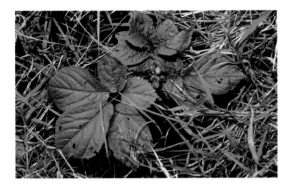

PANAX IS DERIVED from the word panacea, meaning a treatment for all problems. The Chinese, some 5,000 years ago, attributed to ginseng many properties and cures. When taken internally, ginseng acts as a general tonic by stimulating the central nervous system. It encourages the secretion of hormones to improve stamina. The stimulant effect may be used to treat stress and chronic fatigue.

Ginseng has been shown to reduce the blood concentrations of both glucose and cholesterol as well as stimulating resistance to disease. It also has a reputation for being an aphrodisiac.

PARTS USED
❦ Root

DOSAGE
❦ *Take 2 teaspoons (10 ml) of ginseng elixir daily for up to two weeks.*

POTENTIAL BENEFITS
❦ *Stimulates the central nervous system*
❦ *Improves stamina*
❦ *Boosts resistance to infection*
❦ *Reduces blood glucose and cholesterol levels*
❦ *May act as an aphrodisiac*

WARNING: Ginseng should not be used continuously for more than one month. In some cases it may cause headaches.

PARSLEY

Petroselinum crispum

ARSLEY WAS FIRST
recorded in an early
Greek herbal as long
ago as the third
century B.C. It
was used in
ancient Rome
in cooking and
in ceremonies. It
is rich in vitamins A
and C and contains
flavonoids that help to
reduce allergic reactions,
but its main action
appears to be
detoxification.

An internal dose of parsley
can help stimulate the menstrual
process and help relieve menstrual
cramps. Parsley also acts as an effective
diuretic and helps relieve kidney
complaints. It also helps reduce
inflammation of the bladder as well as
the stomach, it can
help relieve colic, flatulence and
indigestion.

The stimulant effect on the uterus
makes this herb one to avoid during
pregnancy, but once the baby is born,
it may help stimulate lactation and
milk flow.

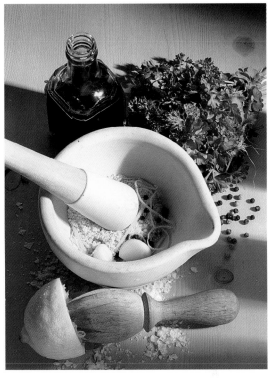

Parsley sprigs can be added to make delicious dressings for salads.

PARTS USED
🌱 *Seeds, leaves, roots and oil extract*

DOSAGE
🌱 *As a liquid tincture, take 20 drops twice daily.*

POTENTIAL BENEFITS
🌱 *Stimulates flow of breast milk*
🌱 *Aids menstrual cramps*
🌱 *Reduces inflammation in the bladder (cystitis)*
🌱 *Stimulates the flow of urine*
🌱 *Helps reduce colic and indigestion*

CULINARY USES
🌱 *Used as an ingredient in sauces and as a garnish for fish, cheese and egg dishes.*
🌱 *Can also be added to dressings and vinaigrettes.*

WARNING: Avoid during pregnancy.

KAVA KAVA

Piper methysticum

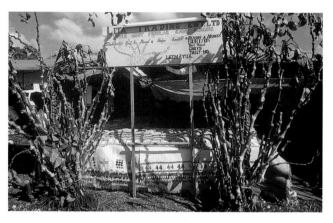

Kava kava dealers on the island of Tonga, Polynesia.

THIS INTOXICATING PEPPER was made into a special drink by the Polynesians and given to Captain Cook. The resulting effects led him to name it botanically as "intoxicating pepper." Kava is still made into a drink by the Melanesians during certain rituals, when it is said to enhance mental awareness.

Herbalists today use this herb to stimulate the nervous and circulatory systems. It cures insomnia and nervousness by enhancing restfulness. Kava kava has the ability to reduce the pain associated with muscle spasms and arthritis.

PARTS USED
❦ *Roots and rhizomes*

DOSAGE
❦ *Take 2 tablets (100 mg) of dried herb daily.*

POTENTIAL BENEFITS
❦ *Acts as a remedy for insomnia*
❦ *Acts as a nerve tonic*
❦ *Acts as a mental stimulant*
❦ *Reduces muscle spasms*
❦ *Helps reduce joint pains associated with rheumatism*

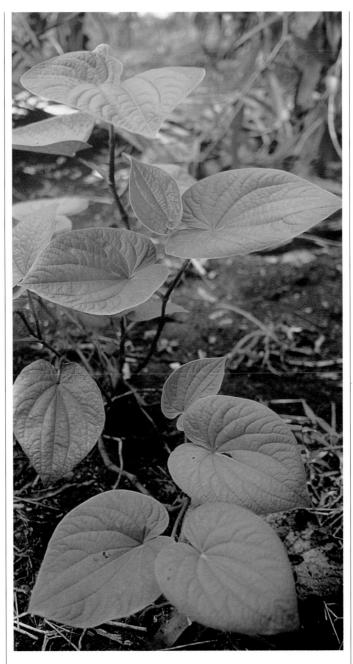

*Kava Kava (*Piper methysticum*)*

GREATER PLANTAIN

Plantago major

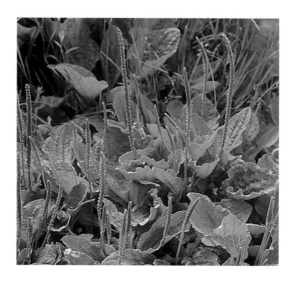

Fᴵʀsᴛ ᴅɪsᴄᴏᴠᴇʀᴇᴅ ɪɴ ancient China in about 206 ʙ.ᴄ., plantain was a popular medicine of the day. Its astringent properties promote healing and act as an effective expectorant in cases of chest infections. These properties led the herb to be used for cases of diarrhea and bowel inflammation. Externally, the juice can be used for ear infections, wounds, inflammation of the eye and hemorrhoids.

Pᴀʀᴛs ᴜsᴇᴅ
❦ *Leaves*

Dᴏsᴀɢᴇ
❦ *As a liquid tincture, take 20 drops twice daily.*
❦ *For external application, crush the leaves and collect the juice, then apply directly to the affected area.*

Pᴏᴛᴇɴᴛɪᴀʟ ʙᴇɴᴇғɪᴛs
❦ *Cleanses wounds*
❦ *Has an antiseptic action*
❦ *Helps control diarrhea and bowel inflammation*
❦ *Reduces ear and eye inflammation*

TORMENTIL OR BLOODROOT

Potentilla tormentilla

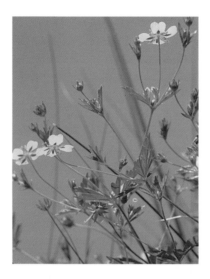

THIS RATHER UNASSUMING plant has very thick and strong roots that, when cut, reveal a blood-red color—hence the common name of bloodroot.

Tormentil contains a high concentration of astringents, making it an important medicinal plant. The action of this herb is mainly due to tannic acid, which makes it a useful preparation for treating diarrhea and inflammatory problems affecting the mucous membranes of the mouth, throat and stomach. Externally, it can be used to help heal wounds and cuts.

PARTS USED
❦ Roots (rhizome)

DOSAGE
❦ As a liquid tincture, take 2 drops twice daily after eating.
❦ For external application, use as a poultice for wounds.

POTENTIAL BENEFITS
❦ Helps treat colitis
❦ Reduces diarrhea
❦ Soothes an irritated throat
❦ Reduces inflammation of the lining of the mouth
❦ Helps heal wounds and cuts

BLACKTHORN

Prunus spinosa

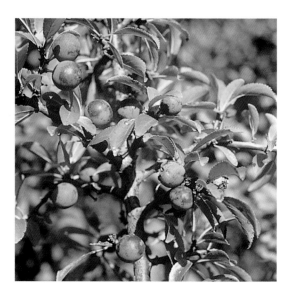

Blackthorn contains very powerful chemicals (anthraquinone glycosides) that stimulate the contraction of the bowel wall, causing nausea, abdominal cramping and vomiting. Storing the herb for a number of years will dramatically reduce this effect.

For this reason, blackthorn has been used as a purgative (to induce vomiting) and, in smaller doses, as a laxative.

PARTS USED
❦ *Bark and fruits*

DOSAGE
❦ *As a liquid tincture, take 20 drops daily.*

POTENTIAL BENEFITS
❦ *Acts as a very effective laxative*
❦ *Acts as a purgative*
❦ *Acts as a diuretic*

WARNING: This herb is very strong. Overdosage will cause vomiting and diarrhea.

ROSEMARY

Rosmarinus officinalis

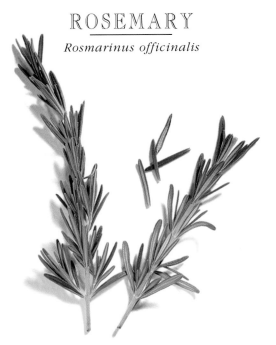

RICH IN volatile oils, rosemary is a very strong antiseptic agent with powerful anti-inflammatory actions. The phenolic acid content of rosemary is responsible for this antimicrobial property. Recent studies have suggested that rosemary may be beneficial in the treatment of toxic shock syndrome, but its historical use as an anti-infective agent is unquestionable.

The internal use of rosemary includes the treatment of depression, fatigue, migraine and tension headaches, poor circulation and digestive disorders including flatulence. Rosemary acts as a good circulatory stimulant and has a balancing and calming effect on the digestive system.

For rheumatism and muscular aches and pains, the external application of rosemary oil can give symptomatic relief. The oil can also be used as an insect repellent and the dried leaves can be used in potpourris and to scent clothes and linen. Traditionally, an infusion of rosemary has been used as a shampoo to stimulate hair growth and as a rinse to lighten blonde hair.

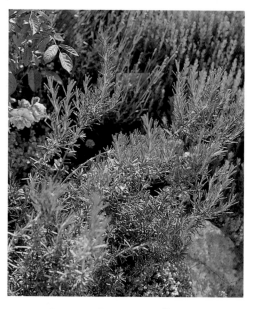

*Rosemary (*Rosmarinus officinalis*)*

PARTS USED
🌿 *Leaves, flowering tips and essential oil*

DOSAGE
🌿 *As an external application, apply 6 drops of essential oil, mixed with 2 teaspoons (10 ml) of almond oil, to the desired area twice daily.*
🌿 *As a liquid tincture, take 10 drops twice daily.*
🌿 *As a tea, add a teaspoon of chopped leaves to 1 cup (250 ml/8 fl oz) of boiling water and let stand for 5 minutes.*

POTENTIAL BENEFITS
🌿 *Acts as an antiseptic agent for cuts and wounds*
🌿 *Has an antidepressant activity*
🌿 *Reduces headache and migraine symptoms*
🌿 *Stimulates circulation and digestion*
🌿 *Relieves flatulence*

CULINARY USES
🌿 *Especially good with lamb and in soups and stews. Leave a fresh sprig in oil to steep for 1 month to produce a flavored oil, that must be refrigerated and used quickly.*

WARNING: The essential oil should not be used internally.

RASPBERRY LEAVES

Rubus idaeus

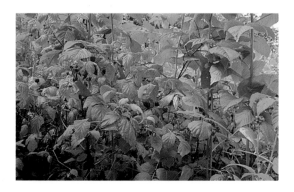

RASPBERRIES HAVE FORMED part of the human diet for as long as fossil records date back; they were even mentioned in the writings of Hippocrates (460–370 B.C.).

The astringent properties of this herb can be of use to pregnant women as it tones up the uterine muscles during pregnancy and is often given in preparation for childbirth. It is also given for a couple of months after birth to help restore the tone of the uterus. As a remedy for menstrual cramps, raspberry tea appears to be very effective.

PARTS USED
❦ *Leaves and fruits*

DOSAGE
❦ *As a tea, add a teaspoon of raspberry leaves (or use a commercial preparation) to 1 cup (250 ml/8 fl oz) of boiling water and drink twice daily during the third trimester of pregnancy.*
❦ *As a remedy for menstrual cramps, sip the tea as needed.*

POTENTIAL BENEFITS
❦ *Aids childbirth labor*
❦ *Tones up the uterus*
❦ *Reduces menstrual cramps*

WARNING: The use of this herb during pregnancy should be restricted to the third trimester.

BUTCHER'S BROOM

Ruscus aculeatus

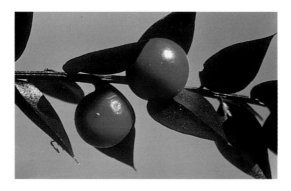

As far back as the first century A.D., butcher's broom was known to have medicinal properties, and it was mentioned as a treatment for kidney stones. Modern techniques have now identified the active agent, a steroid-like substance that can effectively reduce inflammation by constricting the veins.

A popular use for this herb is as a mild diuretic. When butcher's broom is taken internally, the circulatory system benefits from its tonic action, and improvements in poor circulation and hemorrhoids have been reported. An external application can be soothing when applied to hemorrhoids.

PARTS USED
🌾 *Young shoots and roots*

DOSAGE
🌾 *As a liquid tincture, take 15 drops twice daily.*
🌾 *For external application, use as a cream, as required.*

POTENTIAL BENEFITS
🌾 *Acts as a circulatory tonic*
🌾 *Has an anti-inflammatory action*
🌾 *Acts as a mild diuretic to reduce swollen ankles*
🌾 *Helps relieve the pain of arthritis*

WARNING: Avoid in cases of high blood pressure.

WHITE WILLOW
Salix alba

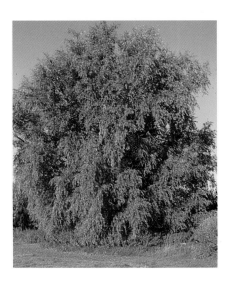

SALIX CONTAINS A natural aspirin-like substance, salicylic acid, which was first produced commercially in 1838. The actions of aspirin are well known and include the reduction of fever, improvement in joint stiffness associated with arthritis and rheumatism, symptomatic easing of headache and reduction of inflammation.

It is interesting to note that pure salicylic acid intake is associated with stomach irritation, but that its presence in the white willow is buffered by tannins, which actually protect the stomach.

PARTS USED
❦ *Leaves and bark*

DOSAGE
❦ *As a liquid tincture, take 20 drops twice daily after eating.*

POTENTIAL BENEFITS
❦ *Acts as an anti-inflammatory agent*
❦ *Helps treat arthritis and rheumatism*
❦ *Reduces fevers*

SAGE

Salvia officinalis

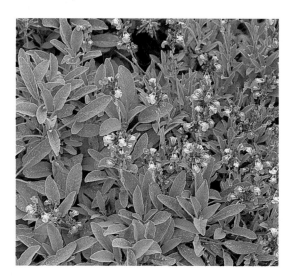

SAGE WAS ASSOCIATED with long life in the eighteenth century and was a cherished herb. A wide array of aromas can be noticed coming from freshly cut sage due to the high content of volatile oils present in the plant.

Sage provides us with a readily available antiseptic agent. Fresh sage juice has anti-inflammatory and antiseptic activities. It can be used as a mouthwash and a gargle for tonsillitis and laryngitis. Sage can be used externally in a compress to promote the healing of wounds.

Sage extracts can effectively relax smooth muscles (found in the internal organs), and it has an effect on the female chemistry rather like that of estrogen. This estrogenic effect can actually reduce and suppress the production of breast milk. Sage can, therefore, be taken to control excessive lactation. The estrogen-like stimulation of sage can help relieve menopausal problems, and sage has been used to assist fertility.

People with indigestion and digestive problems such as dyspepsia benefit from this herb.

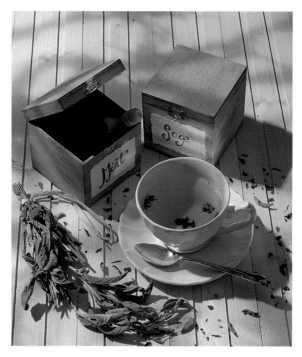

*Sage (*Salvia officinalis*) tea is useful for combating stress.*

PARTS USED
🌿 *Leaves*

DOSAGE
🌿 *As a liquid tincture, take 20 drops twice daily.*
🌿 *For external application, use as a compress for wounds.*

POTENTIAL BENEFITS
🌿 *Stimulates fertility*
🌿 *Helps relieve menopausal problems*
🌿 *Reduces excessive milk production in lactating women*
🌿 *Has antiseptic and anti-inflammatory effects*

CULINARY USES
🌿 *The leaves can be made into a pleasant tea or used in the traditional manner as a key ingredient in stuffings. Sage can also be used as a garnish for vegetable soup. Use sparingly as it is quite strong.*

WARNING: Avoid during pregnancy as large quantities of this herb are toxic.

CLARY

Salvia sclarea

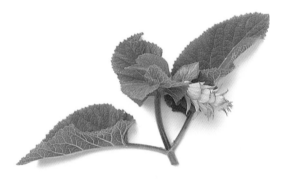

THERE ARE MORE than 750 different species in the sage family. The term "clary sage" (also known as muscatel) is derived from the folkloric words "clear eye."

The volatile oil is used in aromatherapy massage and has many therapeutic actions. It is very effective as an antidepressant. It has a calming effect and can act as a sedative. Clary is also used as a general tonic for the whole body and helps to relieve menstrual cramps. This oil blends very well with sandalwood (*Santalum album*) and lavender (*Lavandula officinalis*), and it is safe to use on children.

PARTS USED
❦ *Essential oil*

DOSAGE
❦ *As an aromatherapy application, use 3 drops in 1 teaspoon (5 ml) of almond oil and massage in the usual way.*

❦ *As a bath for children, add 2 drops in 1 teaspoon (5 ml) of almond oil and mix in the bath.*

POTENTIAL BENEFITS
❦ *Relieves depression*
❦ *Has a calming effect*
❦ *Helps reduce menstrual cramps*

WARNING: Avoid during early pregnancy. Do not use when drinking alcohol.

ELDER

Sambucus nigra

WHEN A COLD is on its way, drink a hot tea made from elder. This will stimulate an increase in body temperature, which will help your body to speed the killing of the invading bacteria or virus. Elder has very effective decongestant properties and can be combined with many herbs to boost their activity in combating chest infections, nasal congestion and chills. This herb can also help relieve hay fever, bronchial congestion and sinusitis. The fruits of elder can be used in relieving rheumatic joint problems.

An external application of elder can be of great relief to irritated skin, bruises, sprains and minor wounds. It can be applied to the skin as an infusion or ointment. Elderflower water can be used as an effective skin toner, lightener and to fade away any unwanted freckles.

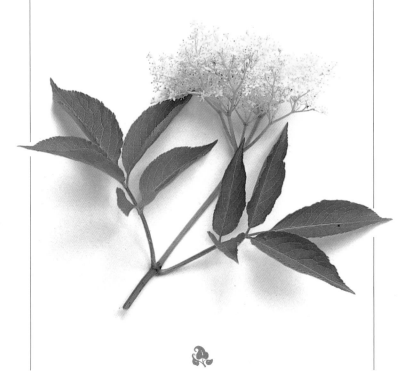

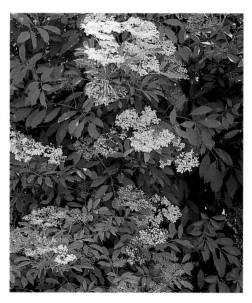

Elder flowers (Sambucus nigra)

PARTS USED
❦ Leaves, bark, flowers and fruits

DOSAGE
❦ A remedy made from elderberry juice boiled with sugar to make a syrup is good taken twice daily for bronchitis and colds.
❦ For external application, use as a cream as required.

POTENTIAL BENEFITS
❦ Helps clear colds and flu
❦ Increases body temperature to assist in the elimination of invading infections
❦ Helps relieve sinusitis
❦ Soothes irritated skin

COSMETIC USES
❦ Can be made into a cleansing milk and lotion to soften the skin

CULINARY USES
❦ Boil the juice from the fruits with a little sugar, ginger and a few cloves to produce elderberry rod (cordial). Preserves and sauces can be made from the fruits.

WARNING: The seeds from the elder can be toxic and should be avoided. Always cook the fruits first before eating them.

SKULLCAP

Scutellaria baicalensis

First mentioned in Chinese writings dating back to 25–220 A.D., skullcap has been used in medicinal preparations ever since. Its active agents such as certain flavonoids that improve liver function make it an important remedy for all kinds of liver disease. Its anti-inflammatory action makes it an effective treatment for poisonous bites, diarrhea and pharyngitis. Skullcap is also used to treat anxiety, depression and insomnia as it relaxes the nervous system.

The plant was used by the Cherokee, to induce menstruation, but this use has now dwindled.

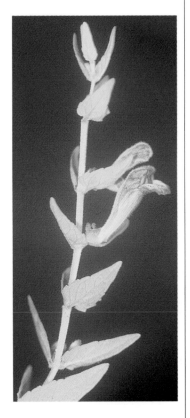

PARTS USED
❧ Roots

DOSAGE
❧ As a liquid tincture, take 20 drops twice daily after eating.

POTENTIAL BENEFITS
❧ Can be used to treat liver disease
❧ Reduces inflammation of stomach and bowel
❧ Reduces diarrhea
❧ Helps cases of sore throat
❧ Can help insomnia

MILK THISTLE

Silybum marianum

T HIS POWERFUL HERB can counteract the damage of a lethal dose of the death cap mushroom (*Amanita phalloides*). Liver enzyme systems are protected by the silymarin content of this bitter herb.

Liver function is not only protected by silymarin, but its function also appears to be enhanced and new liver cells can be seen to appear. This action is used to treat liver cirrhosis and hepatitis, both potentially fatal conditions.

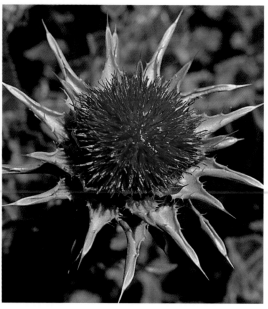

PARTS USED
❦ *Whole plant*

DOSAGE
❦ *As a liquid tincture, take 20 drops twice daily.*

POTENTIAL BENEFITS
❦ *Acts as a powerful liver protector*
❦ *Helps fight hepatitis*
❦ *May help regenerate damaged liver cells*

COMFREY

Symphytum officinale

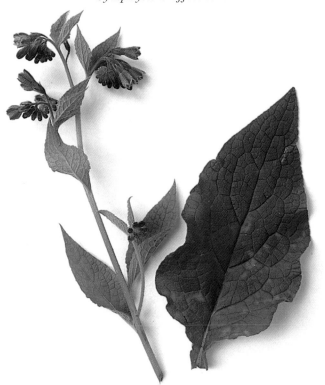

COMFREY IS PROBABLY one of the best-known medicinal herbs. Its use by herbalists can be traced back over many centuries and is related to borage (*Borago officinalis*). Comfrey is known under other names including knitbone as it can heal bone fractures. Recent work has isolated an active agent, a pyrrolizidine alkaloid, which is responsible for the healing actions of comfrey, but this substance can induce liver damage and tumors. For this reason, internal usage is not recommended.

Used externally, comfrey has the ability to speed the healing of wounds and comfrey creams are perfectly safe and are very effective remedies for poorly healing wounds, eczema, psoriasis, hemorrhoids and skin ulcers. A comfrey poultice can be used to help heal sprains and severe cuts and to soothe

soothe pain and inflammation. It can also be used to drain boils and abscesses. Comfrey cream has been used for the treatment of mastitis in nursing women, but, because of its possible toxic effects, this should be avoided in case the infant should ingest some of the cream during feeding.

PARTS USED
❧ Leaves and roots

DOSAGE
❧ For external application, use as a cream locally as required.
❧ For external application use as a poultice as required.

POTENTIAL BENEFITS
❧ Heals skin
❧ Speeds the healing of wounds
❧ Soothes hemorrhoids
❧ Reduces inflammation associated with eczema and psoriasis
❧ Helps drain boils and abcesses
❧ Helps relieve sprains

COSMETIC USES
❧ Add an infusion of comfrey leaves for a healing bath.
❧ May be used in a lotion to soften the skin.

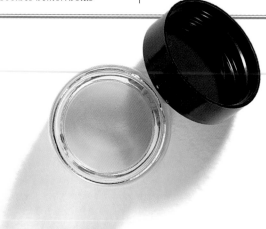

*Comfrey (*Symphytum officinalis*) can be used in lip balm to protect the lips.*

WARNING: Do not take internally or use for the treatment of mastitis if breast-feeding.

CLOVES

Syzygium aromaticum

FRESH CLOVES look quite different from the dark twiglike dried herb we are used to seeing. As far back as 600 A.D., the Chinese were documented to use cloves for many different reasons.

The volatile oil contained in cloves, eugenol, gives them their unique aroma. Another active constituent of cloves, methyl salicylate, has been recently identified and may be involved in the painkilling aspects attributed to clove extracts.

For toothache, clove oil should be used. Apply a small amount either directly on the tooth or use a cotton swab for difficult-to-reach areas. It is not recommended to leave absorbent cotton soaked in clove oil for too long in one place because the surrounding tissue of the mouth may suffer. When taken internally, cloves can help an upset stomach, symptoms of nausea, chills and even impotence.

PARTS USED
❦ *Flower buds and oil*

DOSAGE
❦ *Apply a few drops of oil to a toothache 2 or 3 times a day.*
❦ *Add 6 cloves to an herbal tea and let stand for 5 minutes.*

POTENTIAL BENEFITS
❦ *Helps an upset stomach*
❦ *Relieves chills and colds*
❦ *Acts as a toothache remedy*

CULINARY USES
❦ *Cloves give a special flavor to preserved meats, especially ham. Stud a ham with cloves and wrap well. After a few days the ham will take on a hint of the clove flavor. Whole cloves can be added to an oil base and allowed to steep for a month to produce a flavored cooking oil that should be refrigerated and used shortly. Cloves may also be used in pickling and baking.*

FEVERFEW

Tanacetum parthenium

THERE HAS BEEN much research performed on this powerful herb. Feverfew contains many chemicals, one of which (parthenolide) has the ability to block the action of serotonin, an inflammatory chemical released from special blood cells called platelets. Prostaglandins, hormonelike substances released from white blood cells, can aggravate migraines by affecting the blood circulation to the brain. These actions are blocked by feverfew extracts. Studies have confirmed that feverfew was a migraine cure. Feverfew has the ability to treat minor fevers, rheumatism and arthritis.

PARTS USED
❦ *Leaves and stalks*

DOSAGE
❦ *As a liquid tincture, take 20 drops twice daily.*

POTENTIAL BENEFITS
❦ *Acts as a migraine treatment*
❦ *Helps control minor fevers*
❦ *May be helpful in cases of joint pain and arthritis*

WARNING: Avoid during pregnancy. It is not advised to eat the fresh leaves because these may cause mouth ulcers in sensitive individuals.

TANSY

Tanacetum vulgare

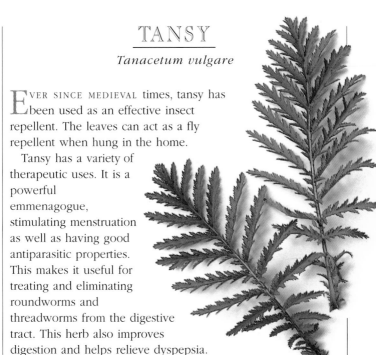

Ever since medieval times, tansy has been used as an effective insect repellent. The leaves can act as a fly repellent when hung in the home.

Tansy has a variety of therapeutic uses. It is a powerful emmenagogue, stimulating menstruation as well as having good antiparasitic properties. This makes it useful for treating and eliminating roundworms and threadworms from the digestive tract. This herb also improves digestion and helps relieve dyspepsia.

Applied externally, tansy can be used to treat scabies as well as help with rheumatism.

Parts used
❦ *Leaves*

Dosage
❦ *For external application, use as a compress to treat scabies and rheumatic joints.*

Potential benefits
❦ *Stimulates menstruation*
❦ *Eliminates worms*
❦ *Improves digestion*
❦ *Relieves dyspepsia*
❦ *Helps treat rheumatism*
❦ *Helps treat scabies*

Culinary uses
❦ *Fresh leaves may be used in salads and egg dishes, but only use in small quantities.*

Warning: Avoid using over a long period of time. Avoid during pregnancy. An overdose of tansy tea or oil can be fatal.

DANDELION

Taraxacum officinale

THE DANDELION FIRST appeared in European medicine in 1480, having been used by the Chinese since 659 A.D.

Dandelion acts as a diuretic, increasing the urine flow so much that early users often called it "wet-the-bed." Its high potassium content is thought to be responsible for this action. High blood pressure has also been reduced by dandelion treatment thanks to its diuretic activity and potassium content.

The liver and gallbladder can benefit from dandelion, which appears to enhance the function of these organs. For this reason it has been used for the treatment of hepatitis, gallstones, gout and skin problems, including eczema.

PARTS USED
❧ Whole plant

DOSAGE
❧ As a liquid tincture, take 20 drops twice daily.

POTENTIAL BENEFITS
❧ Acts as a liver-stimulating agent
❧ Increases flow of bile
❧ Helps in skin conditions such as eczema
❧ Lowers blood pressure
❧ Increases urine flow (diuretic)
❧ Is a good source of potassium

COSMETIC USES
❧ Add an infusion of dandelion leaves to the bath to cleanse the skin.

CULINARY USES
❧ Cook fresh leaves like spinach or add to a salad.

THYME

Thymus vulgaris

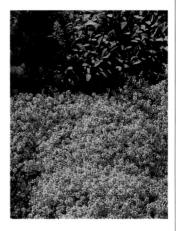

THYME IS ANOTHER herb with valuable antiseptic properties, the active agent being thymol. The aroma of thyme varies among species and depends on the concentrations of oils present in the plant. Thyme is an herb with a long tradition of use in respiratory problems. It is taken internally for coughs and colds or more serious problems such as bronchitis and asthma. The mucus-clearing ability of thyme makes it the appropriate remedy for chronic congestion when inflammation is a problem. Externally thyme can soothe painful joints.

PARTS USED
❦ *Whole plant*

DOSAGE
❦ *As a liquid tincture, take 20 drops twice daily.*
❦ *For external application, use 6 drops of essential oil, mixed with 2 teaspoons (10 ml) of almond oil and apply to the desired area.*

POTENTIAL BENEFITS
❦ *Clears lung congestion and infections*
❦ *Helps reduce asthma symptoms*
❦ *Has an antiseptic action*
❦ *Relieves colds*
❦ *Soothes painful joints*

CULINARY USES
❦ *Thyme is the basis of bouquet garni. Try adding a little to soups, meat and fish dishes. Added to marinades, thyme provides a special flavor.*

WARNING: Do not use the essential oil internally. Avoid during pregnancy.

FENUGREEK

Trigonella foenum-graecum

As FAR BACK as 1500 B.C., fenugreek was being used and its effects documented in the writings of the ancient Egyptians. Its ability to reduce muscular spasm made it the herb of choice in menstrual cramps and labor pains. It was even used in ancient civilizations to induce childbirth.

Modern medicine has been interested in extracts of fenugreek since the isolation of two chemicals: trigonelline, a potential cancer treatment, and certain saponins that can be used in contraceptive preparations.

The traditional use of this herb has been in the treatment of non-insulin-dependent diabetes, inflammation of the stomach, digestive problems and menstrual cramps. Fenugreek is also used to stimulate the flow of breast milk in nursing mothers. An external application can help arthritis.

PARTS USED
❧ *Leaves and seeds*

DOSAGE
❧ *As a liquid tincture, take 20 drops twice daily.*
❧ *For external application, use as a poultice, mix freshly crushed seeds with a little water and apply as needed.*

POTENTIAL BENEFITS
❧ *Reduces menstrual cramps*
❧ *Can stimulate the flow of breast milk*
❧ *Improves digestion*
❧ *Assists in the balance of blood sugars*
❧ *Soothes arthritic joints*

CULINARY USES
❧ *Use fenugreek seeds to add a spicy flavor to pea soups and to cooked carrots.*

COLTSFOOT

Tussilago farfara

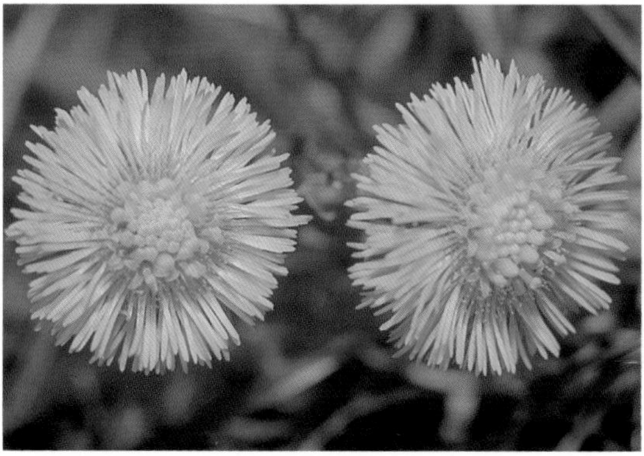

THE PLANT WAS used as far back as 23–79 A.D., when the leaves and roots were burned over coals and the smoke generated was taken as a remedy for persistent cough. During the classical period, coltsfoot was smoked for the treatment of asthma and lung congestion.

Coltsfoot has a licorice flavor. It is used for the control of spasms involving the respiratory system. As a cough expectorant, coltsfoot is quite effective, but its main application is to reduce inflammation associated with irritated mucous membranes in the respiratory tract. Externally, coltsfoot has a soothing effect on inflamed skin, especially eczema and dermatitis.

PARTS USED

- *Flowers and leaves*

DOSAGE

- *As a liquid tincture, take 20 drops twice daily after eating.*
- *For external application, use as a compress for eczema and dermatitis.*

POTENTIAL BENEFITS

- *Acts as a cough remedy and expectorant*
- *Helps control asthma*
- *Eases symptoms of bronchitis and laryngitis*
- *Has a soothing effect on inflamed skin*

SASSAFRAS LEAVES

Umbellularia californica

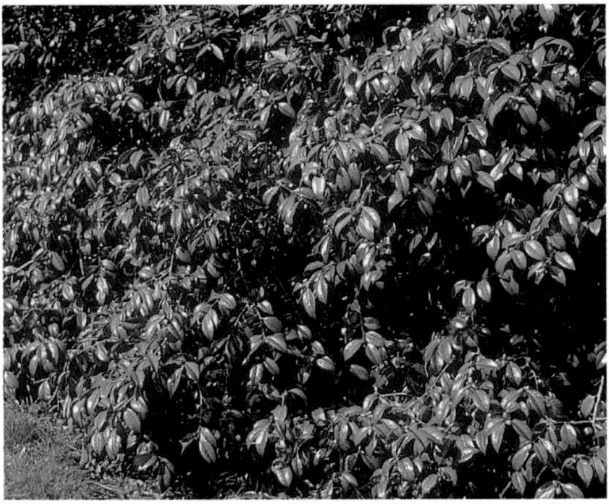

A NATIVE PLANT of California, sassafras leaves were found to be a very effective insect repellent. The sassafras plant has a strong camphoraceous aroma, and it has been used as an inhalant for the treatment of headaches and sinus congestion. The leaves have been used traditionally for the treatment of headache and neuralgia, for which they are bound to the painful area in the form of a poultice.

PARTS USED
- *Leaves*

DOSAGE
- *As an infusion, take 2 or 3 cups (475–750 ml/16–25 fl oz) daily.*
- *As a liquid tincture, take 25 drops twice daily.*

POTENTIAL BENEFITS
- *Acts as a headache remedy*
- *Helps in cases of neuralgia*

CULINARY USES
- *Try using in place of bay leaves in meat dishes or stews.*

WARNING: Do not use sassafras roots as they are carcinogenic.

NETTLE

Urtica dioica

NETTLE HAS BEEN used since Roman times for treating rheumatic disease. The Romans would flail the inflamed joints with nettles to induce an inflammatory reaction that would calm down the disease.

Nettles contain a rich source of nutrients, especially vitamins A, B and C, and minerals including silica. The astringent properties of the herb can help reduce the blood flow, control bleeding and reduce blood pressure. It may be used to treat nosebleeds.

Taken internally, nettles can help rebalance the nutritional status of anemia sufferers. It may be helpful in controlling excessive menstrual bleeding. Arthritis, gout and rheumatism can all be reduced by using nettles, probably due to their diuretic action.

PARTS USED
❦ *Whole plant and leaves*

DOSAGE
❦ *As a liquid tincture, take 20 drops twice daily.*

POTENTIAL BENEFITS
❦ *Reduces symptoms of arthritis and rheumatism*
❦ *Supports requirements needed to prevent anemia*
❦ *Controls bleeding*

COSMETIC USES
❦ *Use in shampoo to help reduce dandruff.*

CULINARY USES
❦ *Cook the young leaves like spinach or purée for soups. Nettles can be made into wine or beer. Older leaves can be gritty and should not be used for cooking.*

WARNING: Do not use the uncooked plant for culinary purposes as it is poisonous and can produce kidney damage.

CRANBERRY

Vaccinium macrocarpon

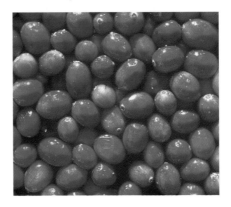

A RECENT REPORT on cranberries estimated their current usage in the United States to be about 400 million pounds (81.5 million kg), which equates to a value of $1.25 billion. Cranberries are certainly popular!

Cranberries contain about 80 percent water and have a high vitamin C content. Their citric acid levels are very high—higher even than that of lemons.

The healing properties of cranberries date back to the seventeenth century, when they were used for the treatment of

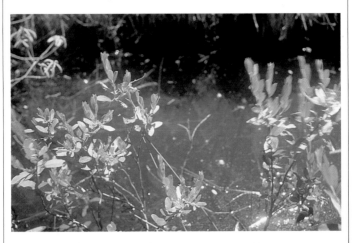

*Cranberry (*Vaccinum macrocarpon*)*

stomach and liver problems. Cranberries have become the herb of choice for the treatment of bladder infections. Studies have located a natural polymer, arbutin, that actually prevents the bacteria from sticking to the wall of the bladder and urinary tract. An earlier theory suggested that cranberries made the urine acidic, which killed bacteria, but this theory has been replaced by the finding that bacteria actually lose their foothold on the walls of the urinary system in the presence of cranberry extracts.

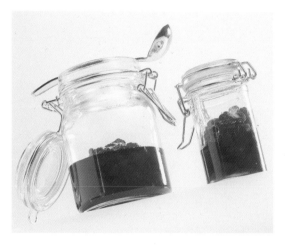

Cranberries are delicious added to preserves.

PARTS USED
🌿 Fruits

DOSAGE
🌿 Take 2 tablets (100 mg) of dried berries twice daily in acute phase, reducing to 1 tablet (50 mg) over the following month.
🌿 Drink 1 teaspoon (5 ml) of cranberry powder (commercially prepared) in ⅔ cup (150 ml/¼ pint) of water twice daily until symptoms ease, reducing to ½ teaspoon (2.5 ml) for the next month.

POTENTIAL BENEFITS
🌿 Acts as a cystitis treatment
🌿 Acts as a urinary cleanser

CULINARY USES
🌿 The fruits can be added to preserves, desserts and salads.

BILBERRY

Vaccinium myrtillus

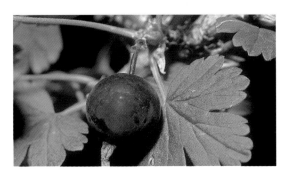

BILBERRY IS FULL of beneficial phytochemicals. Blood sugar levels are improved by the substances known as glucoquinones, while other agents called anthrocyanosides keep blood circulation flowing by dilating blood vessels. The species of bilberry *Vaccinium myrtillus* contains a unique substance (arbutin) that has powerful antiseptic effects on the urinary system and has been used as an effective natural cystitis treatment.

During World War II, Royal Air Force pilots in the United Kingdom received preserves made from bilberry to improve their night vision. It is interesting to note that recent studies have confirmed that bilberry extract can regenerate visual purple (the chemical that keeps night vision healthy) and, therefore, improve vision.

PARTS USED
❦ *Leaves and fruits*

DOSAGE
❦ *As a liquid tincture, take 20 drops twice daily.*

POTENTIAL BENEFITS
❦ *Improves vision*

❦ *Stabilizes blood sugar levels*
❦ *Acts as an effective cystitis remedy*

CULINARY USES
❦ *Bilberry preserves is a common product. The fruits may be added to salads and incorporated into desserts.*

VALERIAN
Valeriana officinalis

THE NAME VALERIAN is derived from the Latin word *valere* meaning "to be well." This herb gives us the opportunity to get well by inducing a restful sleep and relaxation, allowing the body to divert its healing powers to where they are most needed.

The traditional uses of this herb include treating hysteria, cramps, indigestion, high blood pressure, painful menstruation, palpitations and, of course, insomnia.

Valerian may be combined with passionflower (*Passiflora incarnata*) for a deeper sedative action, or it can be combined with licorice (*Glycyrrhiza glabra*) or hyssop (*Hyssopus officinalis*) and used as a cough expectorant. This herb can also help treat mouth ulcers when used as a mouthwash.

PARTS USED
❦ *Rhizome, roots and oil extract*

DOSAGE
❦ *As a sleep aid, take 25 drops of liquid tincture at bedtime.*
❦ *As a mouthwash, use a cooled infusion.*

POTENTIAL BENEFITS
❦ *Acts as a calming agent*
❦ *Induces a restful sleep*
❦ *Helps in panic attacks*
❦ *Reduces muscular tension*
❦ *Aids in menstrual cramps*

MULLEIN

Verbascum thapus

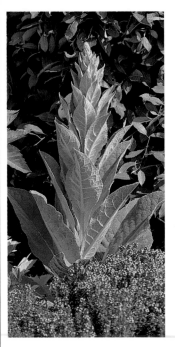

MULLEIN HAS BEEN used in folkloric medicine to treat respiratory disorders including coughs, congestion, and asthma. It was traditionally used to treat serious wasting conditions such as tuberculosis and was associated with witchcraft. It was thought that witches used the hairs on top of the leaves to make potions. The stems were also dipped in tallow and used as torches by the Greeks and Romans. Mullein has good expectorant and anti-inflammatory properties and can be used to soothe dry and irritating coughs as well as help expel phlegm.

PARTS USED
❦ *Leaves*

DOSAGE
❦ *As an infusion, add 2 teaspoons (10 ml) of dried leaves to 1 cup (250 ml/8 fl oz) boiling water and let stand for 5 minutes.*
❦ *Take a liquid tincture made from the flowers for coughs and sore throats.*
❦ *Take a leaf tincture for eliminating phlegm.*

POTENTIAL BENEFITS
❦ *Soothes dry and irritated coughs*
❦ *Acts as a mild sedative*
❦ *Has a mild diuretic action*
❦ *Has an expectorant action*
❦ *Has an anti-inflammatory action*

COSMETIC USES
❦ *Use the dried flowers infused in water to make a hair rinse to lighten hair.*

VERVAIN

Verbena officinalis

VERVAIN HAS A long history of medicinal uses, especially treating nervous disorders.

Taken internally, vervain can help depression that is often present after an illness and can help treat stress-related headaches and migraines.

This herb contains bitters that stimulate the liver and help relieve hepatitis and jaundice. It also stimulates the digestive system and improves digestion. Vervain has a diuretic action, which makes it useful for relieving fluid retention. This herb is an effective emmenagogue. Taken as a tea at bedtime, it acts as a mild sedative.

Vervain can be used to soothe inflamed eyes. This herb can also be used to treat insect bites and sprains.

PARTS USED
🌿 *Leaves*

DOSAGE
🌿 *As a tea, add 2 teaspoons of dried leaves to 1 cup (250 ml/ 8 fl oz) of boiling water and let stand for 5 minutes before drinking.*
🌿 *For external application, use as a diluted infusion for soothing inflamed eyes.*
🌿 *For external application, use as a poultice for insect bites and minor injuries.*

🌿 *For external application, use as an ointment for eczema.*

POTENTIAL BENEFITS
🌿 *Helps depression*
🌿 *Improves digestion*
🌿 *Alleviates nervous disorders*
🌿 *Helps relieve hepatitis and jaundice*
🌿 *Stimulates menstruation*
🌿 *Has a diuretic action*
🌿 *Has a mild sedative action*
🌿 *Helps soothe inflamed eyes*

WARNING: Avoid during pregnancy as vervain acts as a stimulant to the uterus.

CRAMPBARK

Viburnum opulus

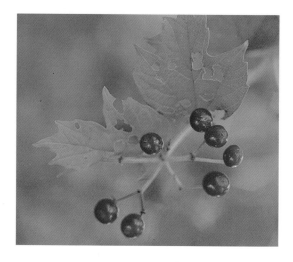

CRAMPBARK AND ITS close relative stagbush (*Viburnum prunifolium*) have been used since colonial times as treatments for painful menstruation. Contained within the plant are botanical substances that relax the uterus and, therefore, reduce the pains associated with menstrual cramps. The plant has also been used in cases of threatened miscarriage and high blood pressure.

PARTS USED
❦ Bark

DOSAGE
❦ *As a liquid tincture, take 20 drops twice daily.*

POTENTIAL BENEFITS
❦ *Reduces pains associated with menstruation and uterine cramps*
❦ *May help prevent miscarriage*
❦ *Helps lower high blood pressure*

WARNING: Do not eat the uncooked fruits as they are poisonous.

YUCCA
Yucca gloriosa

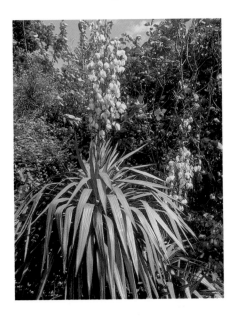

THE CHEMICAL SAPONIN contained within the yucca has been shown to affect toxins absorbed by the stomach bacteria. It is these toxins that may be responsible for the destruction of joint cartilage, so yucca, in blocking the uptake, may hold possible therapeutic applications in the treatment of arthritis. This observation has been supported by the traditional use of yucca by Native Americans for the treatment of inflamed joints and rheumatism.

PARTS USED
❦ Sap

DOSAGE
❦ *Take 2 tablets (100 mg) of dried sap daily.*

POTENTIAL BENEFITS
❦ *Reduces inflammation*
❦ *Eases symptoms of rheumatism*
❦ *May be a possible arthritis remedy*

GINGER

Zingiber officinale

GINGER'S ACTIVE AGENT is gingerol. It was a curious observation that dried ginger was more pungent than the fresh root. It turns out that upon drying, gingerols broke down into chemicals called shogaols, which are twice as potent.

Ginger's main effect on humans is to reduce nausea and motion sickness. It has become a popular herb for the treatment of morning sickness associated with pregnancy. Its safety in recommended doses is good, but excessive intake can be dangerous. This herb also promotes gastric secretions and is useful in treating flatulence.

Ginger has been used as a traditional treatment for skin irritations, both externally applied and by internal dosage.

For colds and flu, ginger extract has a warming effect and can boost the immune response to infection. Ginger has a powerful diaphoretic action and induces sweating. It can also be used as a gargle to relieve sore throats.

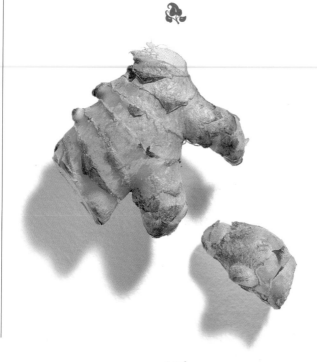

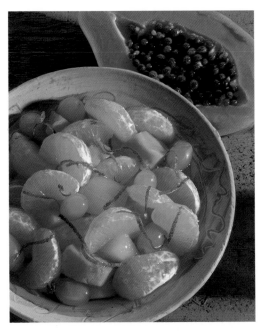

*A ginger (*Zingiber officinale*) dressing is a delicious accompaniment to fruit.*

PARTS USED

❦ *Rhizome and oil extract*

DOSAGE

❦ *As a liquid tincture, take 25 drops twice daily.*
❦ *As a tea, crush a slice of fresh gingerroot and add to the infusion.*

POTENTIAL BENEFITS

❦ *Acts as an antinausea remedy*
❦ *Helps in morning sickness*
❦ *Reduces cold and flu symptoms*
❦ *Induces sweating*
❦ *Helps relieve flatulence*
❦ *Boosts the immune response*

CULINARY USES

❦ *Add a couple of slices of freshly chopped gingerroot to a stir-fry, curry or gingerbread mixture for an extra-fresh flavor, or add to salad dressings.*
❦ *To make a ginger dressing, put ½ cup (50 g/2 oz) of sugar and ⅔ cup (150 ml/¼ pint) of water in a saucepan and heat gently, stirring, until the sugar has dissolved. Bring to a boil, then simmer 1 minute without stirring. Remove from the heat and add ⅔ cup (150 ml/¼ pint) of ginger wine, two pieces of chopped stem ginger, finely grated rind and juice of 1½ limes. Pour over fruit and leave to cool. Chill before serving.*

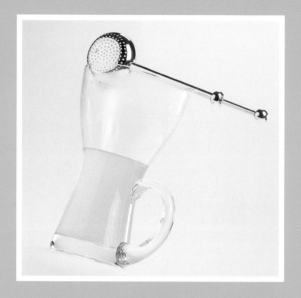

REMEDIES

HERBAL REMEDIES FOR CHILDREN

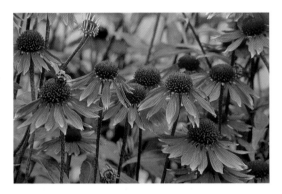

*Echinacea (*Echinacea purpura*) helps stimulate the immune system.*

Fever

It is important to remember that a fever is not always a bad thing, but keeping a close watch on the child's temperature is important. The average body temperature is 98.6°F (37.0°C). A lower temperature is suggestive of shock or excessive cooling if you are sponging your child down with cold water, or it could be a sign that the temperature is going to increase soon, possibly up to 103°F (39.8°C) or more. Temperatures up to 101°F (38.8°C) are thought of as moderate fever; when this rises to 102° to 104°F (39.2–40.3°C) or more, it is considered to be seriously high, and prompt medical attention is strongly advised.

Basic natural methods are often enough to help your child through most fevers of the mild to moderate variety. If your child has a fever but is not sweating, try to stimulate sweating by using a natural sweat-inducing agent (known as a diaphoretic).

A hot tea made from elder (*Sambucus nigra*) or

Sweat-Inducing Formulation

Make a decoction using 2 tablespoons (30 ml) to 2¼ cups (500 ml/18 fl oz) of water. This tea is taken hot, about 1 or 2 cups (250–475 ml/8–16 fl oz), along with a warm-hot bath.

chamomile (*Anthemis nobilis*) has a considerable stimulatory effect and can break a fever very effectively.

During the entire illness, doses of echinacea (*Echinacea purpura*) should be given at regular intervals to assist in the stimulation of the immune system. Its antiviral and antibacterial properties are other factors that make this the best extract for all illnesses.

Upset Stomach and Diarrhea

All children from time to time suffer from a nonspecific infection and other maladies that tend to induce acute diarrhea and stomach pains often accompanied by a mild fever.

Other causes of upset stomachs in children include food poisoning, new food in the diet (often rich foods), overexcitement and fright, very cold or chilled foods, overeating, too much sun and mental or physical distress.

For diarrhea, try a tincture of dandelion (*Taraxacum officinalis*) or tormentil (*Potentilla tormentilla*). Caution: Diarrhea can be life-threatening. So, if the diarrhea does not appear to improve and the child is becoming dehydrated, seek urgent medical attention. As the upset stomach slowly improves, the appetite may take a little while to return to normal; if this is the case, try a dose of centaury (*Centaurium erythraea*).

Rehydration Formulation

Boil a scant 1 cup (200 ml/ 7 fl oz) of water, and, as it cools, add 1 teaspoon (5 ml) of sugar, a generous pinch of baking soda and a smaller pinch of salt. Stir until all of the ingredients have dissolved and give to the child when the formula is cold.

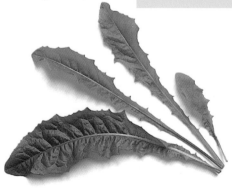

Common Childhood Diseases

Chicken pox This condition is also known as *Varicella* and is one of the most contagious diseases known today.

For the symptoms of skin irritation, try an application of aloe vera (*Alo barbadensis*) salve or chamomile (*Anthemis nobilis*) lotion. Taking a tea made from yarrow (*Achillea millefolium*), chamomile (*Anthemis nobilis*) or goldenseal (*Hydrastis canadensis*) can be beneficial. A tincture of echinacea (*Echinacea purpura*) should always be taken.

Common Cold There is no cure for the common cold, but by using naturopathic principles, it should be possible to control many symptoms and, with luck, prevent your child from catching colds regularly. A daily dose of echinacea is essential, along with plenty of vitamin–C-rich foods. Supplements are advised if your child is fussy about eating fruits and vegetables. If there is a persistent cough, try sage tea, or for excessive mucus, a tea made from fenugreek (*Trigonella foenum-graecum*) or ginger (*Zingiber offinale*) can be very effective. A tincture of goldenseal (*Hydrastis canadensis*) is advisable during the infectious period to assist in fighting the infection.

A tea made from ginger, fennel and honey is an ideal remedy for colds.

Measles Natural supportive measures include using tinctures of yarrow (*Achillea millefolium*) and echinacea (*Echinacea purpura*). A tea made from yarrow, with the addition of a few drops of echinacea tincture, can be very beneficial. To stimulate the appetite when the worst of the disease is over, try a tincture of barberry (*Berberis vulgaris*).

Mumps There is no specific treatment for mumps, but the glands will settle within 10 days. General naturopathic measures should be followed.

Eczema and Psoriasis

It is interesting that eczema and psoriasis share some key factors. Both skin conditions are aggravated by stress and anxiety. The underlying reason for this is not known, but stress does increase the levels of certain hormones known to stimulate the circulation to the skin, which inflames an already irritated condition. The second common factor lies in the observation that essential fatty acid metabolism and the metabolism of micronutrients such as selenium and zinc appear to be defective.

The irritation can be related to an imbalance in inflammatory chemicals, such as histamines, and dry flakiness. Raised patches of skin occur due to an excessive production of deeper skin layers that rapidly migrate to the surface. Unfortunately, the trigger mechanisms behind such changes are, at present, unknown. Some claim that dietary allergy or chemical contact can start these changes, and in some sufferers, this is definitely the case, but in most there is a coexistent nutritional imbalance. Selenium and zinc, as well as other micronutrients, are needed for healthy skin cell maturation. A corrective daily dose of the nutrients zinc and selenium taken for a month, followed by a lower dose of these minerals for another month or so, should rebalance this situation.

Skin inflammation is best approached by optimizing fatty acid metabolism. There are many essential fatty acids, but the most important to the skin appear to be gamma linoleic acid (GLA) and the omega 3 and 6 oils.

Derived from borage (*Borago officinalis*) seed and evening primrose (*Oenothera biennis*) seeds, GLA is probably the best known of all the essential fatty acids. The only all-natural source of GLA is breast milk, which may go some of the way to explaining the link between eczema and bottle-fed babies. The omega 3 and 6 oils are found in fish and fish oils, linseeds, marine algae and meat from marine mammals such as seals and whales. Flaxseed (*Linum usitatissimum*) oil contains both GLA and the omega 3 and 6 oils in one balanced form.

An interesting herb known as *Plectranthus barbatus* or sometimes *Coleus forskohlii* is showing great promise as a remedy for psoriasis. It is best taken as a dried extract in commercially prepared tablet or capsule form.

Asthma and Hay Fever

It is unfortunate, but both of these distressing conditions appear to go hand in hand. Both may be based in allergies, usually to inhaled triggers, but they may have other aggravating factors such as food sensitivities.

An elimination diet is the most sensible course of action to take when investigating food allergies, but this method is best followed under professional supervision to ensure that a balanced diet is maintained during the testing process.

Herbal remedies such as Chinese skullcap (*Scutellaria baicalensis*), licorice (*Glycyrrhiza glabra*), garlic (*Allium sativum*) and angelica (*Angelica archangelica*) commonly feature in the management of childhood asthma and hay fever.

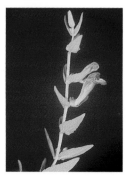

Chinese skullcap
(*Scutellaria baicalensis*)

Garlic (*Allium sativum*) has the ability to prevent a special enzyme (lipoxygenase) from working. The enzyme activates an important part of the inflammatory response, which is prevented by supplementation with garlic extract.

Angelica (*Angelica archangelica*) is especially effective in those individuals suffering from allergies to pollen, dust and animal dander. These allergens play an important role in generation of symptoms in hay fever and asthma.

Licorice (*Glycyrrhiza glabra*) also has anti-inflammatory and anti-allergy activity with a cortisone-like action. Steroids are widely used in the long-term management of asthma. Licorice extract has none of the side effects of steroids, but it does have many of the benefits. The inflammatory aspect of asthma can be managed using this extract.

Chinese Skullcap (*Scutellaria baicalensis*) has been used for its anti-inflammatory properties in the management of arthritis for many years. The herb contains high levels of flavonoids that work in a similar way to some anti-asthmatic drugs.

Common Problems and Remedies

COLIC

- Extract of dill
  (*Anethum graveolens*)
- Fennel water
  (*Foeniculum vulgare*)
- Tincture of ginger
  (*Zingiber officinale*)
- Tincture of cloves
  (*Syzygium aromaticum*)

CONSTIPATION

- Extract of licorice
  (*Glycyrrhiza glabra*)
- Tincture of barberry
  (*Berberis vulgaris*)

COUGH

- Elder syrup (*Sambucus nigra*)
- Tincture of plantain
  (*Plantago major*)
- Tea made from marshmallow
  (*Althaea officinalis*)

COUGH WITH PHLEGM

- Tincture of echinacea
  (*Echinacea purpura*)
- Tea made from ginger
  (*Zingiber officinale*) and fennel
  (*Foeniculum vulgare*) with
  honey

CRADLE CAP

- Tincture of burdock
  (*Arctium lappa*)
- Tincture of nettle
  (*Urtica dioica*)
- Tincture of dandelion
  (*Taraxacum officinale*)
- Plantago ointment
  (*Plantago major*)
- Olive oil (*Olea europaea*)

DIAPER RASH

- Zinc and castor oil cream
- Calendula ointment
  (*Calendula officinalis*)

EARACHE

- Tincture of hops
  (*Humulus lupulus*)
- Tincture of St. John's wort
  (*Hypericum perforatum*)
- Tincture of goldenseal
  (*Hydrastis canadensis*)
- Tincture of echinacea
  (*Echinacea purpura*)
- Tincture of plantain
  (*Plantago major*)

NASAL CONGESTION

- Tea made from hyssop
  (*Hyssopus officinalis*)
- Tincture of hyssop
  (*Hyssopus officinalis*)
- Tincture of goldenseal
  (*Hydrastis canadensis*)
- Extract of garlic
  (*Allium sativum*)

SLEEPING PROBLEMS

- Tincture of lemon balm
  (*Melissa officinalis*)
- Tea made from lemon balm
  (*Melissa officinalis*)
- Tincture of valerian
  (*Valeriana officinalis*)
- Tincture of hops
  (*Humulus lupulus*)

SORE THROAT

- Tincture of marshmallow
  (*Althaea officinalis*)
- Tincture of plantain
  (*Plantago major*)
- Tincture of elder
  (*Sambucus nigra*)
- Tincture of echinacea
  (*Echinacea purpura*)

TEETHING

- Tincture of chamomile
  (*Anthemis nobilis*)
- Marshmallow syrup
  (*Althea officinalis*)

HERBAL REMEDIES FOR YOUNG PEOPLE AND ADULTS

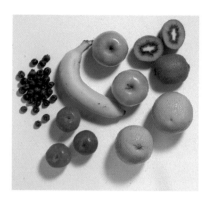

Premenstrual Syndrome (PMS)

Tension is probably one of the most common symptoms reported by women who suffer from a menstrual dysfunction. It has been estimated that up to 75 percent of women suffer from some form of premenstrual anxiety. Other symptoms such as food cravings, weight gain and depression also occur to varying degrees. There are many safe, natural ways to conquer PMS that do not have dangerous side effects.

Anxiety is a common problem. This tends to be due to a hormone imbalance, namely excessive estrogen and low progesterone levels. The high estrogen has a blocking effect on vitamin B6, inhibiting the liver production of serotonin and altering the ability to balance blood sugar levels. A rise and fall of sugars is partly responsible for mood elevation and depression.

Herbal extracts of dandelion root (*Taraxacum officinalis*) contain the plant chemical inulin (not to be confused with the hormone insulin), which has a balancing effect on blood glucose levels. This can be used alongside the trace mineral chromium to help control fluctuating sugar levels associated with premenstrual problems.

Depression is suffered by about 30 percent of women with PMS. This might be an effect of disordered brain chemistry (namely, serotonin) or a dysfunction of other brain chemicals.

The exact cause is not known, but there appears to be a link with estrogen levels. The extract from St. John's wort (*Hypericum perforatum*) is very effective at relieving this type of depression. In one study, more than 65 percent of those treated improved while using St. John's wort extract. The active agent, hypericin, was standardized in these tests.

It is not uncommon for women to gain more than 3 pounds (1.4 kg), mostly due to water retention. The hormone to blame is aldosterone, which appears in excess in the premenstrual phase of the cycle, again linked to the estrogen imbalance. A dose of uva-ursi (*Arctostaphylos uva-ursi*) taken from the time of ovulation (day 14 of the cycle) will increase the urine flow and control fluid retention.

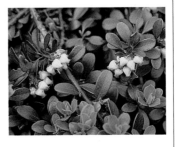

*Uva-ursi (*Arctostaphylos uva-ursi*)*

Natural Considerations Adjust the types of food to include complex carbohydrates such as pasta, potato and rice and reduce the intake of animal fats. Eat simpler foods such as vegetables and fruit.

The essential fatty acids contained in evening primrose oil can help with menstrual cramps and pain as well as help to balance hormone levels. A dose of 500–1,000 mg taken at bedtime with water is recommended.

Substances such as feverfew extract (*Tanacetum parthenium*) have been able to stop prostaglandins from being produced, and this is important for those who suffer menstrual discomfort.

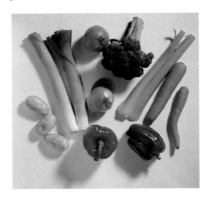

Cystitis

Cystitis is a common problem. Most cases are due to an infection traveling up from the vagina into the bladder. Flare-ups often occur after sexual intercourse, when the infection is reintroduced into the bladder.

Cystitis in men results from an infection traveling to the bladder from the urethra or from the prostate gland, which may itself be harboring a bacterial infection. The most common symptoms in both men and women are pain and urgency—a constant sensation of the need to pass urine. Blood may be passed in the urine indicating the severity of the bladder infection. It is important to remember that the infection can travel up from the bladder into the kidneys and this requires urgent medical treatment.

Three-Step Treatment for Cystitis

For most people, the following steps can be followed, and a successful treatment for cystitis can be achieved.

Step 1 Increase fluid intake. Few people drink enough water to keep themselves hydrated. We lose about 6¼ cups (1.5 liters/2½ pints) of water daily through our breath, sweat, urine and feces, so to remain in balance, you need to drink that amount daily. This does not take into account activity levels that cause us to sweat, body type, temperature, food consumption, stress levels etc. As a rule, 8 cups (2 liters/3⅓ pints) of water (preferably bottled water) are recommended.

Step 2 Try to locate, or better still, make, unsweetened cranberry (*Vaccinium macrocarpon*) juice and drink 2 cups (475 ml/16 fl oz) daily. Cranberry powders and capsules are available. The dose for powders is 2 teaspoons (10 ml) taken in the morning and evening or two capsules taken twice daily. If you cannot obtain unsweetened cranberry juice, take the capsules or powders. Increasing your sugar intake will just encourage excessive bacterial growth in the bladder.

Step 3 Increase general health and boost immunity. It is advisable to check that your diet contains the correct balance of foods. Taking echinacea (*Echinacea purpura*) extract has been shown to elevate white blood cell activity and stimulate the immune response. Take 25–30 drops of liquid extract twice daily or take 2 capsules twice daily.

Irritable Bowel Syndrome (IBS)

It has been estimated that more than half of the abdominal problems are diagnosed as IBS. Because it is common, you may think there is a simple cure, but in a case of IBS you need to take a holistic view of health in order to plan an individual treatment program. Each sufferer may have similar symptoms, but it is not uncommon to find different aggravating factors ranging from food sensitivities to stress.

One popular theory suggests that there is an imbalance in the body's nervous system. A specialized division of the nervous system (the autonomic nervous system) controls the internal running of our bodies such as the beating of the heart, and plays a vital role in the coordinated activity of the digestive system. The stomach and bowels are at work 24 hours a day digesting food, absorbing water and nutrients, killing invading bacteria and collecting waste matter. This activity needs to be controlled on a subconscious level, leaving the brain free to conduct day-to-day business.

In times of stress, the body brings the "fight-or-flight" mechanism into play. During this, we prepare ourselves, biologically, to fight or run away from danger. In either case, adrenaline is released, and nervous activity is stimulated. The bowel cannot contract and move normally and symptoms such as abdominal bloating, pain and cramping, fatigue, alternating bouts of constipation and diarrhea, passage of mucus in the stool, flatulence and nausea are common. Another common finding is that the pain of IBS is often relieved by the passing of stools while some find that certain foods induce the pain.

It is important to seek professional advice when bowel symptoms are experienced, since other conditions may mimic IBS—conditions such as lactose intolerance, celiac disease, diverticular disease and bowel cancer. These conditions have their own special collections of symptoms that must be ruled out before IBS can be diagnosed.

IBS needs an individual treatment program, but some guidelines can be followed that may give relief.

Dietary Fiber Increasing the intake of soluble dietary fiber from vegetables, fruits, oat bran, beans and psyllium husk can be beneficial. However, this must be done slowly since the bowel in IBS tends to be hyperactive and may respond unfavorably with an unaccustomed dose of fiber.

Bowel Spasms For the symptomatic control of bowel spasms, the use of peppermint (*Mentha piperita*) oil capsules offers relief. Peppermint oil has relaxing effect on the smooth muscle that forms the bowel wall. Capsules that are coated pass through the stomach undigested and open up in the lower bowel. Generally, 0.2-ml capsules are used at doses of two or three capsules taken between meals.

Other antispasmodic agents are the herbs valerian (*Valeriana officinalis*), rosemary (*Rosmarinus officinalis*), chamomile (*Anthemis nobilis*) and lemon balm (*Melissa officinalis*).

Diarrhea When diarrhea and irritation are the main symptoms, an old preparation called Robert's formula has survived. It combines marshmallow (*Althaea officinalis*) root, cabbage (*Brassica oleracea*) extract, echinacea (*Echinacea purpura*), goldenseal (*Hydrastis canadensis*), okra (*Hibiscus esculentis*) and slippery elm (*Ulmus fulva*) to produce a remedy for the bowels. Modern preparations of Robert's formula are available in capsules and should be taken at a dose of one or two capsules between meals.

Nausea The nausea experienced by sufferers may be helped by taking ginger (*Zingiber officinale*). Studies have documented how effective ginger can be in treating motion sickness and

---

Ingredients in Robert's Formula

❦

Cabbage extract
(*Brassica oleracea)* 100 mg

Marshmallow root
(*Althaea officinalis*) 100 mg

Okra
(*Hibiscus esculentis*) 75 mg

Slippery elm
(*Ulma fulva*) 75 mg

Echinacea
(*Echinacea purpura*) 25 mg

Goldenseal
(*Hydrastis canadensis*) 25 mg

nausea. Ginger used in cooking or taken as a dietary supplement will not upset sensitive bowels, and it may calm the spastic nature of IBS as well as reduce the nausea.

Psychological Aspects Finally, the psychological aspects of IBS must not be forgotten. Almost all sufferers complain of fatigue, anxiety, depression, feelings of hostility or sleep disturbances. These problems need attention and can be overcome with the correct help.

Common Problems and Remedies at a Glance

ACNE
- Tincture of echinacea
  (*Echinacea purpura*)
- Tincture of goldenseal
  (*Hydrastis canadensis*)
- Tincture of dandelion
  (*Taraxacum officinalis*)

CANDIDIASIS
(Yeast infection)
- Tincture of goldenseal
  (*Hydrastis canadensis*)
- Tincture of echinacea
  (*Echinacea purpura*)
- Extract of garlic
  (*Allium sativum*)

CHRONIC FATIGUE
- Tincture of echinacea
  (*Echinacea purpura*)
- Tincture of goldenseal
  (*Hydrastis canadensis*)
- Licorice root extract
  (*Glycyrrhiza glabra*)
- Extract of panax or Siberian
  ginseng (temporary measure
  only) (*Panax ginseng*)

HYPERTENSION
- Extract of garlic
  (*Allium sativum*)
- Tincture of hawthorn berry
  (*Crataegus oxyacantha*)
- Tincture of mistletoe
  (*Viscum alba*)

INFLAMMATORY BOWEL DISEASE
- Marshmallow root extract
  (*Althaea officinalis*)
- Extract of cabbage
  (*Brassica oleracea*)
- Tincture of echinacea
  (*Echinacea purpura*)
- Tincture of goldenseal
  (*Hydrastis canadensis*)
- Extract of slippery elm
  (*Ulmus fulva*)

MIGRAINE
- Tincture of valerian
  (*Valeriana officinalis*)
- Tincture or extract of feverfew
  (*Tanacetum pathenium*)

OBESITY
- Tea made from dandelion
  (*Taraxacum officinalis*)

SINUS INFECTIONS
- Tincture of echinacea
  (*Echinacea purpura*)
- Tincture of goldenseal
  (*Hydrastis canadensis*)

SPORTS INJURIES
- Extract of turmeric
  (*Curcuma longa*)
- Witch hazel ointment
  (*Hamamelis virginiana*)

HERBAL REMEDIES FOR PREGNANT AND BREAST-FEEDING WOMEN

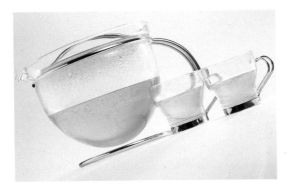

> **WARNING:** No pregnant woman should take any preparation without consulting with her health-care practitioner.

Morning Sickness

There have been many ideas to help explain morning sickness, but the trigger is still shrouded in mystery.

Teas made from fennel (*Foeniculum vulgare*), peppermint (*Mentha piperita*) or ginger (*Zingiber officinale*) can give relief from symptoms. Taking a nighttime cup of chamomile (*Anthemis nobilis*), lemon balm (*Melissa officinalis*) or hops (*Humulus lupulus*) tea will help you get a restful sleep. There has been suggestions that ginger may be toxic during pregnancy, but all of the reviews state that the intake obtained via a tea is safe. The problem can arise when multiple concentrated extracts are taken in capsule or tablet form.

Emotional Problems

During pregnancy, moods may swing, and emotions become unbalanced. It is important to relax and have a good soak in a warm bath using a few drops of essential oils. Lavender (*Lavandula officinalis*) and chamomile (*Anthemis nobilis*) oil can be very relaxing. A tincture of rosemary (*Rosmarinus officinalis*) can also help.

Heartburn

As the baby grows, it will take up a lot of space within your lower abdomen. This causes the stomach to become pushed up, and its contents occasionally leak into the lower part of the food pipe causing heartburn. Attention to diet is vital, as is taking digestive aids such as dill *(Anethum graveolens)* or caraway *(Carum carvi)*. These can be chewed or made into a tea and sipped during or between meals. Powdered slippery elm bark *(Ulmus fulva)* can give relief from the irritation of stomach acid.

Varicose Veins and Hemorrhoids

To prevent these, you will need to include garlic *(Allium sativum)* in daily meals to keep the circulation strong. Try a tea made from dandelion *(Taraxacum officinalis)*. Extracts of St. John's wort *(Hypericum perforatum)* can be made into a tea and taken two or three times daily.

To strengthen the walls of the veins, drink a tea made from fresh ginger *(Zingiber officinale)*. If the skin is irritated, try making a compress from comfrey *(Symphytum officinale)* and marshmallow *(Althaea officinalis)*, plantain *(Plantago major)*. For an intensive treatment of hemorrhoids that may be bleeding, apply a comfrey cream directly to the area.

Lactation

Remedies used to encourage the flow of breast milk have been used for centuries and do offer help. Infusions of milk thistle *(Silybum marianum)*, nettle *(Urtica dioica)*, fenugreek *(Trigonella foenum-graecum)* and hops *(Humulus lupulus)* are all safe to use during this time. These herbs may also help reduce the risk of colic in the baby.

Mastitis

If caught early, this condition can be reversed without antibiotics. As soon as mastitis is suspected, express your milk by hand or use a breast pump, and take a dose of flaxseed *(Linum usitatissimum)* oil, 1–3 tablespoons (15–45 ml) daily. If there is no improvement within 48 hours, seek medical advice.

Sore Nipples

The application of comfrey *(Symphytum officinale)* cream has been questioned by those who consider that accidental intake

Herbs to Avoid in Pregnancy

Yarrow
(Achillea millefolium)

Angelica
(Angelica archangelica)

Camomile
(Anthemis nobilis)

Celery
(Apium graveolens)

Bearberry
(Arctostaphylos uva-ursi)

Arnica
(Arnica montana)

Wormwood
(Artemisia absinthium)

Southernwood
(Artemisia abratanum)

Calendula
(Calendula officinalis)

Gotu kola
(Centella asiatica)

Black cohosh
(Cimicifuga racemosa)

Myrrh
(Commiphora molmol)

Eyebright
(Euphrasis officinalis)

Fennel
(Foeniculum vulgare)

Licorice
(Glycyrrhiza glabra)

Goldenseal
(Hydrastis canadensis)

Hyssop
(Hyssopus officinalis)

Juniper
(Juniperus communis)

Devil's claw
(Martynia annua)

Nutmeg
(Myristica fragrans)

Pennyroyal
(Mentha pulegium)

Sweet marjoram
(Origanum majorana)

Parsley
(Petroselinum crispum)

Poke root
(Phytolacca americana)

Raspberry leaves
(Rubus idaeus)

Rye
(Ruta graveolens)

Sage
(Salvia officinalis)

Clary
(Salvia sclarea)

Feverfew
(Tanacetum parthenium)

Tansy
(Tanacetum vulgare)

Thuja
(Thuja occidentalis)

Thyme
(Thymus vulgaris)

Vervain
(Verbena officinalis)

of the cream from the nipple when feeding the baby is dangerous. Keeping in mind its long history and the lack of reports of toxic reactions, there is little risk, but if you wish to avoid this cream, use a yarrow *(Achillea millefolium)* -based cream. Do not use yarrow if you are pregnant.

HERBAL REMEDIES FOR MENOPAUSE SYMPTOMS

It has been reported that up to 75 percent of women suffer unpleasant menopause symptoms due to decreasing levels of hormones. For the majority, the symptoms may be short-term (lasting for two to three years), but for others they may persist for more than five years, making life intolerable.

Menopause symptoms are likely to occur at about 50 years of age, unless surgery (hysterectomy) brings on symptoms earlier. Over this transition, menstruation usually becomes irregular until it stops altogether. Menopause is a normal and natural phase of a woman's life, and for many it can herald the start of a special era. With the family grown up, attention can be focused on the woman—so long as she feels well!

Emotions may alter, and the person may become more forgetful. The sleep pattern could change, especially if night sweats are troublesome. Other symptoms may include hot flashes; joint stiffness; vaginal dryness; loss of sexual interest; anxiety; recurrent urinary tract infections; changes in hair, nail and skin quality; and loss of self-esteem.

Many of these problems are short-term, but other symptoms may not appear until much damage has been done. These include osteoporosis and the effects of heart disease and elevated blood cholesterol.

Look very carefully at diet and learn a little about some very interesting plant extracts that have a phytoestrogen activity (an estrogen-like activity but extracted from a plant) in the body. Foods naturally high in phytoestrogens include soy, fennel (*Foeniculum vulgare*), celery (*Apium graveolens*), parsley (*Petroselinum crispum*), flaxseed oil (*Linum usitatissimum*), nuts and seeds. Because of this alternative activity, such herbal extracts are often prescribed for hormone-excess conditions (premenstrual syndrome) as well as hormone-deficiency problems (menopause).

A high-dose vitamin E and C supplement can be of great help. It has been shown that vitamin E helps reduce hot flashes and vaginal problems compared to placebo treatment.

Many herbs have been used in traditional folk medicine as uterine tonics, formulated to relieve menopause symptoms. The classic example is black cohosh *(Cimicifuga racemosa)*, but licorice *(Glycyrrhiza glabra)*, chaste berry *(Vitex anguscastus)* and ginseng *(Panax ginseng)* are considered to be good sources as well.

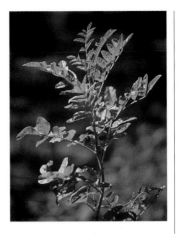

Licorice (Glycyrrhiza glabra*)*

Black cohosh has a history of use dating back to when Native Americans used it as a remedy for menstrual cramps and menopause symptoms. Studies have concluded that the plant has an estrogen-like effect by virtue of its ability to rebalance hormone levels.

Historically, licorice has been used for the treatment of feminine disorders, an application that is now supported by scientific research, which can confirm a mild estrogen-like activity.

Panax ginseng (also known as Korean ginseng) was viewed as a masculine "tonic" until its estrogen-like activity was demonstrated. This action can be so strong that in high doses, the extract may induce postmenopausal bleeding.

The following daily formulas are recommended as part of a natural treatment program. Use one or the other.

Formulas for Menopause
❦

Formula 1
Licorice extract
(Glycyrrhiza globra) 25 mg
Black cohosh
(Cimicifuga racemosa) 25 mg
Chaste berry extract
(Vitex anguscastus) 25 mg
Fennel seed extract
(Foeniculum vulgare) 12 mg

Formula 2
Vitamin E 150 IU
Flaxseed oil
(Linum usitatissimum) 300 mg
Gamma-oryzanol 100 mg

HERBAL REMEDIES FOR THE ELDERLY

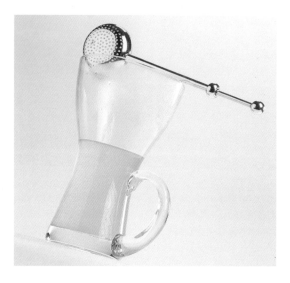

Arthritis

There are many types of arthritis; some result in extreme inflammation and joint deformity, while others cause long-term pain, stiffness and a less severe degree of joint deformity. Osteoarthritis is the most common type of joint condition. The underlying process is one of joint degeneration whereby the smooth joint coverings lose their ability to provide frictionless motion. The cartilage starts to develop patches where its surface has become eroded. This acts as a focus for more erosion, and what was once a small patch soon expands into a much larger area of degeneration. The visible signs of arthritis are a thickening of the tissue and the appearance of nodules around the edges of the joint.

Natural diuretic herbs can

> ### *Golden Grass Tea (Dried Herb)*
> ❧
>
> 40% Goldenrod
> *(Solidago virguaria)*
> 30% *Betula alba*
> 15% Birch
> *(Polygonum avicularea)*
> 10% Horsetail
> *(Equisetum arvense)*
> 5% Pansy *(Viola tricolor)*

help in the elimination of toxic substances such as uric acid by increasing the flow of urine. The two formulas listed below have a safe and effective action on the kidneys, and they are best combined with a special herbal tea, known as golden grass tea.

Formulas for Arthritis

Formula 1 (tincture)

50% Goldenrod
(Solidago virguaria)
14% Silverweed
(Potentilla anserina)
13% Birch
(Betula alba)
5% *Ononis spinosa*
5% Pansy
(Viola tricolor)
5% *Polygonum aviculare*
4% Horsetail
(Equisetum arvense)
4% Juniper
(Juniperus communis)

**Formula 2
(solid extracts)**

Bearberry
(Arctostaphylos Uva-ursi) 100 mg
Lespedeza capitatae 50 mg
Boldo
(Peumus boldo) 50 mg
Goldenrod
(Solidago virguaria) 50 mg

To support the elimination process and assist in the reduction of inflammation, a combination herbal tincture remedy can be very effective.

Massage given by a qualified therapist can be a great relief when applied to the muscle structures that surround the degenerated joint. Massage increases circulation, aids in the drainage of tissue fluids and stimulates the release of healing substances. Aromatherapy can also be helpful. Useful aromatherapy oils for arthritis include eucalyptus *(Eucalyptus globulus)*, ginger *(Zingiber officinale)*, lavender *(Lavandula officinalis)* and rosemary *(Rosmarinus officinalis)*.

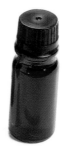

A selection of massage oils

Common Problems
and Remedies at a Glance

It is recommended that you consult a health-care professional before
embarking on a program of self-treatment.

ALZHEIMER'S DISEASE
- Tincture or capsules of ginkgo
  (*Ginkgo biloba*)

ANGINA
- Tincture or capsules of
  hawthorn (*Crataegus
  oxyacantha*)

ATHEROSCLEROSIS
- Extract of garlic
  (*Allium sativum*)
- Extract of alfalfa
  (*Medicago sativa*)
- Tincture or capsules of ginger
  (*Zingiber officinale*)

BRONCHITIS
- Extract of licorice (*Glycyrrhiza
  glabra*)
- Tincture of echinacea
  (*Echinacea purpura*)
- Extract of garlic
  (*Allium sativum*)

DIABETES
- Extract of aloe vera
  (*Alo barbadensis*)
- Extract of bilberry
  (*Vaccinium myrtillus*)

- Extract of fenugreek
  (*Trigonella foenum-graecum*)
- Extract of garlic
  (*Allium sativum*)
- Tincture or capsules of ginkgo
  (*Ginkgo biloba*)
- Tincture of burdock
  (*Arctium lappa*)
- Tincture of dandelion
  (*Taraxacum officinalis*)
- Tincture of artichoke
  (*Cynara scolymus*)

GLAUCOMA
- Tincture or capsules of gingko
  (*Gingko biloba*)

PROSTATE DISEASE
- Tincture of nettle
  (*Urtica dioica*)

VARICOSE VEINS
- Extract of bilberry (*Vaccinium
  myrtillus*)
- Tincture or capsules of ginkgo
  (*Ginkgo biloba*)
- Tincture of horse chestnut
  (*Aesculus hippocastanum*)
- Tincture of hawthorn
  (*Crataegus oxyacantha*)

Herbal Tincture

15% *Polygonum aviculare*
15% Goldenrod
(*Solidago virguaria*)
10% Butterbur (*Petasites officinale*)
10% Silverweed
(*Potentilla anserina*)
10% Yarrow (*Achillea millefolium*)

10% Birch (*Betula alba e foliu...*)
10% Mistletoe (*Viscum alba*)
10% Horsetail
(*Equisetum arvense*)
5% *Colchicum autumnale*
5% Peppermint
(*Mentha piperita*)

HERBAL REMEDIES
FOR TIMES OF STRESS

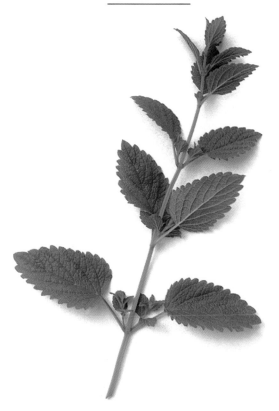

Herpes Simplex and Cold Sores

There is no sign like an eruption of cold sores to indicate that the body is under stress. The immune system becomes suppressed, and opportunistic diseases such as herpes simplex make their appearance.

Lemon balm *(Melissa officinalis)* has been known as an herbal remedy for more than 2,000 years. During the 1960s, the dried extract was reported to exhibit antiviral activity in a number of studies. The efficiency of cream containing lemon balm depends on starting the therapy within eight hours of the onset of symptoms. And to be effective, the cream needs to be very concentrated, containing a 70:1 lemon balm extract with 1 percent allantoin.

Common Problems and Remedies at a Glance

EXHAUSTION
- Tincture of oats (*Avena sativa*)
- Extract of ginseng
  (*Eleutherococcus senticosus*)

FATIGUE
- Tincture or tablets of hyssop
  (*Hyssopus officinalis*)
- Extract of ginseng
  (*Eleutherococcus senticosus*)

HEADACHE
- Tincture of valerian
  (*Valeriana officinalis*)
- Extract of butterbur
  (*Petasites hybridus*)

HIGH BLOOD PRESSURE
- Tincture of mistletoe
  (*Viscum alba*)
- Extract of garlic
  (*Allium sativum*)

INSOMNIA
- Tincture of passionflower
  (*Passiflora incarnata*)
- Tincture or capsules of valerian
  (*Valeriana officinalis*)

IRRITABILITY
- Tincture of oats
  (*Avena sativa*)
- Tincture of lemon balm
  (*Melissa officinalis*)
- Tincture of hops
  (*Humulus lupulus*)
- Tincture of valerian
  (*Valeriana officinalis*)
- Tincture of passionflower
  (*Passiflora incarnata*)

MIGRAINE
- Extract of butterbur
  (*Petasites hybridus*)
- Tincture of lemon balm
  (*Melissa officinalis*)

PALPITATIONS
- Tincture of hawthorn
  (*Crataegus oxyacantha*)
- Tincture of passionflower
  (*Passiflora incarnata*)

POOR MEMORY
- Tincture or capsules of ginkgo
  (*Ginkgo biloba*)

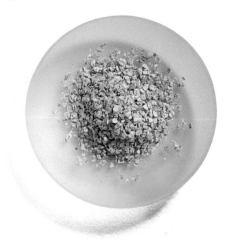

HERBAL REMEDIES FOR EMOTIONAL PROBLEMS

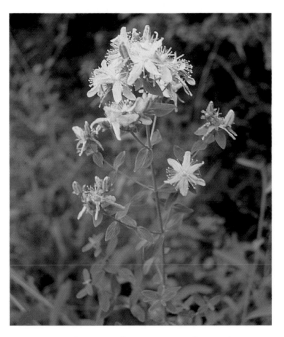

St. John's wort (Hypericum perforatum*)*

Depression

It has been estimated that nearly one in four people experiences some degree of depression at some time in their lives, with women tending to be at a slightly higher risk than men. The biochemistry of mood and mood disturbance is complex, but it is known that many nutritional and environmental factors play a vital role in psychological health. There has been no single factor identified as the cause of depression.

An herbal substance that shows promise in the battle against depression is St. John's wort (*Hypericum perforatum*). This shrubby plant is native to Europe and has been used medicinally for centuries. Studies in Germany have found that the active agent, hypericin, alters brain chemistry and improves mood. Hypericin appears to be able to increase the brain's production of dopamine, an effect similar to many prescription drugs dispensed for depression. Other studies have shown that a standardized extract of St. John's wort is more effective than prescription antidepressants such as amitriptyline that are associated with significant side effects. The use of St. John's wort does not lead to any significant side effects.

The dose of St. John's wort taken in these studies was 300 mg (containing 0.125% hypericin). St. John's wort preparations are available in 300-mg capsules (standardized to contain 0.3% hypericin) and should be taken at the dose of two to three capsules daily.

Other herbs that may help in this condition include ginkgo *(Ginkgo biloba)* and Siberian ginseng *(Eleutherococcus senticosus).*

Common Problems and Remedies at a Glance

ANXIETY

❦ Extract of kava kava *(Piper methysticum),* as needed
❦ Extract of Korean ginseng *(Panax ginseng),* as needed

PANIC ATTACKS

❦ Valerian *(Valeriana officinalis)* capsules, as needed

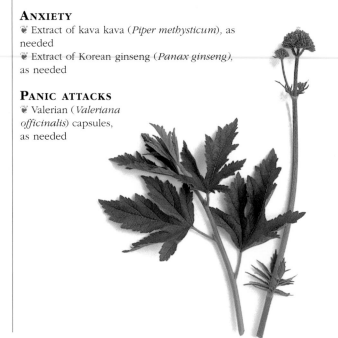

HERBAL FIRST AID KIT

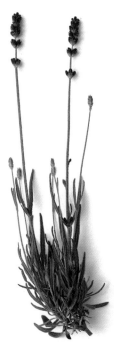

Keeping an accessible collection of essential natural remedies around the house will encourage their use over their potentially more toxic pharmaceutical counterparts. The first aid kit can include bandages, arnica liniments, scissors, herbal-based creams, essential oils and gels. The following chart shows what you need in the basic first aid kit.

Basic First Aid Kit

Echinacea (*Echinacea purpura*) tincture or capsules
Arnica (*Arnica montana*) and comfrey (*Symphytum officinale*) creams
Arnica tincture or tablets
Essential oils: tea tree (*Melaleuca alternifolia*), chamomile (*Anthemis nobilis*) and lavender (*Lavandula officinalis*)
Ginger (*Zingiber officinale*) capsules or tablets
St. John's wort (*Hypericum perforatum*) oil
Aloe vera (*Alo barbadensis*) gel

USING HERBS
IN A BUSY LIFE

It is an unfortunate fact of life that most of us lead hectic lifestyles and, as much as we would like to slow down, the pressures of day-to-day living forbid it! Herbal medicine can help keep our bodies in balance.

Growing herbs for home use can be great fun and an enjoyable hobby, but the preparation of medicines—although possible at home—needs much time and effort, especially if you need to maintain a home supply of medicinal remedies for regular use.

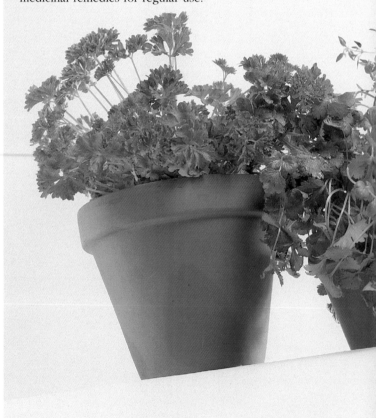

For this reason, the use of prepared tinctures and encapsulated dried extracts has become a popular alternative to the home production of medicinal remedies. The herbs listed in the following section, Recommended Over-the-Counter Remedies, are available worldwide as single-tincture preparations or as combination remedies. Most are developed

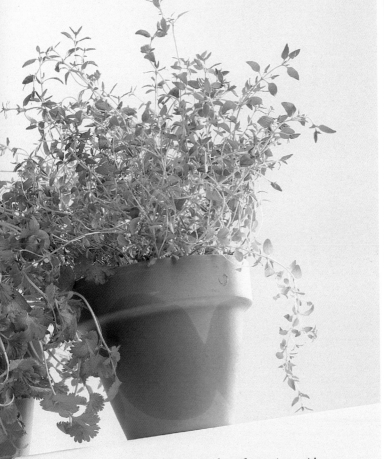

according to strict production codes of practice, with organically grown herbs prepared to a pharmaceutical grade, but always read the label carefully. Using such remedies allows the user to maintain their remedy intake while minimizing the fuss of home production.

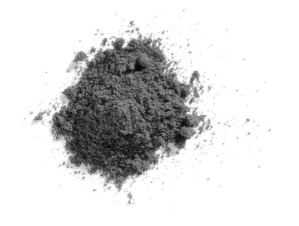

RECOMMENDED OVER-THE-COUNTER REMEDIES

Each remedy listed will support and stimulate the itemized function or system, and in the case of vaginal thrush *(Candida albicans),* the aim is to eliminate the condition.

ADRENAL FUNCTION
❧ Korean ginseng
(Panax ginseng)
❧ Siberian ginseng
(Eleutherococcus senticosus)
❧ Licorice *(Glycyrrhiza glabra)*

BLADDER HEALTH
❧ Cranberry
(Vaccinium macrocarpon)
❧ Uva-ursi
(Arctostaphylos uva-ursi)

BOWEL FUNCTION
❧ Fenugreek
(Trigonella foenum-graecum)
❧ Ginger *(Zingiber officinale)*
❧ Marshmallow
(Althea officinalis)
❧ Peppermint *(Mentha piperita)*

EYE FUNCTION
❧ Bilberry *(Vaccinium myrtillus)*

HEART AND CIRCULATION
❧ Cayenne pepper
(Capsicum frutescens)
❧ Garlic *(Allium sativum)*
❧ Ginkgo *(Ginkgo biloba)*

HORMONE (FEMALE) FUNCTION
❧ Fennel seed
(Foeniculum vulgare)
❧ Licorice *(Glycyrrhiza glabra)*

HORMONE (MALE) AND PROSTATE FUNCTION
❧ Ginkgo *(Ginkgo biloba)*
❧ Korean ginseng
(Panax ginseng)

IMMUNE SYSTEM
❧ Echinacea
(Echinacea purpura)
❧ Goldenseal
(Hydrastis canadensis)

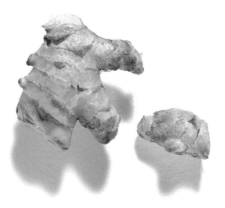

JOINTS
- Butterbur *(Petasites hybridus)*
- Horsetail *(Equisetum arvense)*
- Peppermint *(Mentha piperita)*
- Yarrow *(Achillea millefolium)*

KIDNEY FUNCTION
- Uva-ursi extract
  (Arctostaphylos uva-ursi)
- Boldo extract *(Peumus boldo)*
- Goldenseal extract
  (Hydrastis canadensis)
- Horsetail *(Equisetum arvense)*
- Juniper
  (Juniperus communis)

LIVER FUNCTION
- Boldo *(Peumus boldo)*
- Dandelion
  (Taraxacum officinale)
- Licorice *(Glycyrrhiza glabra)*
- Peppermint *(Mentha piperita)*

LUNG FUNCTION
- Fenugreek
  (Trigonella foenum-graecum)
- Garlic *(Allium sativum)*
- Marshmallow
  (Althaea officinalis)
- Thyme *(Thymus vulgaris)*

LYMPHATIC SYSTEM
- Goldenseal
  (Hydrastis canadensis)

NERVOUS SYSTEM
- Chamomile
  (Anthemis nobilis)
- Hops *(Humulus lupulus)*
- Passionflower
  (Passiflora incarnata)
- Valerian
  (Valeriana officinalis)

SKIN HEALTH
- Chamomile
  (Anthemis nobilis)
- Horsetail
  (Equisetum arvense)
- Rosemary
  (Rosmarinus officinalis)
- Sage *(Salvia officinalis)*

VAGINAL THRUSH
- Goldenseal
  (Hydrastis canadensis)
- Oregano
  (Origanum vulgare)
- Peppermint
  (Mentha piperita)
- Thyme *(Thymus vulgaris)*

GLOSSARY

Addison's disease – disease caused by the underactivity of the adrenal glands

Adrenal glands – glands situated just above the kidneys

Adrenaline – hormone secreted by the adrenal gland that is released in response to physical and mental stress and initiates a variety of responses, including increasing the heart rate

Analgesic – relieves pain

Anemia – deficiency of hemoglobin in the blood

Antiallergy – reduces allergic reactions

Antibacterial – prevents the formation of bacteria

Antibiotic – prevents the growth of bacteria

Antidepressant – alleviates depression

Anti-inflammatory – reduces inflammation

Antimicrobial – destroys pathogenic microorganisms

Antiseptic – prevents the growth of bacteria

Antispasmodic – relieves muscle spasms or cramps

Aphrodisiac – increases sexual desire

Aromatherapy – therapeutic use of essential oils usually through massage

Bacteriostatic – prevents the growth of bacteria

Bitters – herbs that have a bitter taste that stimulate the appetite and aid digestion

Carminative – relieves flatulence and settles the digestive system

Cholagogic – stimulates the flow of bile into the intestine

Cicatrisant – promotes the healing of skin and formation of scar tissue

Colic – abdominal pain in the intestines

Cortisone-like action – reduces inflammation

Cystitis – inflammation of the bladder

Decongestant – helps eliminate nasal congestion

Diaphoretic – promotes sweating

Diuretic – stimulates the secretion of urine

Douche – application of liquid into the vagina

Dyspepsia – indigestion

Elixir – tincture with added sugar or syrup

Emmenagogue – stimulates menstruation

Essential oils – base materials in aromatherapy that are highly aromatic and volatile and are produced from plants by means of extraction, usually distillation

Expectorant – helps to expel mucus and relieves congestion in the digestive tract

Flatulence – large amounts of gas in the stomach and intestines

Flavonoid – substance responsible for the colors yellow and orange in herbs, fruit and vegetables

Histamine – substance released in response to allergic reactions

Holistic – approach that considers the patient's body, mind and spirit

Lactation – secretion of breast milk

Laxative – promotes the evacuation of the bowels

Mastitis – acute inflammation of the breasts

Mucilage – viscous liquid that forms a protective layer over the mucous membranes and skin

Nervine – a nerve tonic, it calms the nerves

Neuralgia – acute nerve pain

Osteoporosis – loss of bone tissue

Phlegm – mucus secreted by the respiratory tract

Pleurisy – inflammation of pleural membrane that surrounds the lungs

Rhizome – underground rootlike structure used as a food store by plants during the winter

Saponin – substance that forms a lather when mixed with water that is found in a variety of herbs and has a wide range of therapeutic properties

Sedative – relieves nervousness and induces sleep with a calming effect

Serotonin – hormone released from the pituitary gland in the brain

Sinusitis – inflammation of the sinuses

Tonic – herbs to strengthen and invigorate a specific organ, system or the whole body

Volatile – evaporates very easily when exposed to air

USEFUL ADDRESSES

Organizations

United Kingdom
Bioforce (UK)
Olympis B Park
Dundonald
Ayrshire, KA2 9BE

**British Naturopathic
Association**
Frazer House
6 Netherhall Gardens
London, NW3 5RR

**The British Herb
Growers Association**
c/o NFU
Agriculture House
London, SW1X 7NJ

**Hadley Wood Healthcare
Ltd. (UK)**
67A Beech Hill
Hadley Wood
Barnet
Herts, EN4 0JW

**Herbal Medicine
Association (UK)**
Field House
Lyle Hole Lane
Redhill
Avon, BS18 7TB

The Herb Society
134 Buckingham Palace Rd.
London, SW11 4RW

Herbal Suppliers
Enzymatic Therapy (UK)
P.O. Box 74
Potters Bar
Herts, EN6 5ZZ

**National Institute of
Herbal Medicine**
9 Palace Gate
Exeter, Devon, EX1 1JA

Naturopathic & Herbal Schools and Universities
**British College of Naturopathy
& Osteopathy**
Frazer House
6 Netherhall Gardens
London, NW3 5RR

Neals Yard Remedies (UK)
1A Rossiter Rd.
London, SW12 9RY

**Power Health Products
(UK)**
10 Central Ave.
Airfield Estate
Pocklington
York, YO4 2NR

Swiss Health Products (UK)
Auchenkyle
Southwoods
Troon
Ayrshire, KA9 1RY

United States of America

American Association of Acupuncture and Oriental Medicine
1424 16th St., NW,
Suite 501
Washington, DC 20036

American Botanical Council
P.O. Box 201660
Austin, TX 78720
512-331-8868

American Herb Association
P.O. Box 1673
Nevada City, CA 95959

Bastyr University
144 N.E. 54th St.
Seattle, WA 98105
206-523-9585

Bioforce (USA)
P.O. Box 507
Kinderhook, NY 12106
518-758-6060

Enzymatic Therapy (USA)
825 Challenger Dr.
Green Bay, WI 54311
414-469-1313

National College of Naturopathic Medicine
11231 S.E. Market St.
Portland, OR 97216
503-255-7355

Canada

Enzymatic Therapy (Canada)
8500 Baxter Place
Burnaby, BC
V5A 4T8

Australia

National Herbalists Association of Australia
Box 65
Kingsgrove, NSW 2208

Short Correspondence (Non-Professional) Courses

United Kingdom

Nutrition with Herbal Medicine
The Edison Institute of Nutrition (UK)
P.O. Box 74
Potters Bar
Herts, EN6 5ZZ

United States of America

Nutrition with Herbal Medicine
The Edison Institute of Nutrition (USA)
2675 W. Highway 89A
Suite 1062
Sedona, AZ 86336

Canada

Nutrition with Herbal Medicine
The Edison Institute of Nutrition (Canada)
2 Bloor St. W. Suite 100
Toronto, Ont. M4W 3E2

INDEX

Bold type indicates a summary of treatment for the condition.